THE CANDIDA CURE

THE CANDIDA CURE

The 90-Day Program to Balance Your Gut, Beat Candida, and Restore Vibrant Health

ANN BOROCH, CNC

Foreword by David Perlmutter, MD

HARPER WAVE

An Imprint of HarperCollins*Publishers*

This book is intended to serve only as a resource and educational guide. This book and the ideas, programs, and suggestions within are not intended as a substitute for the medical advice of physicians. The reader should regularly consult a physician in matters relating to his or her health and particularly with respect to any symptoms that may require diagnosis or medical attention. Neither the author nor the publisher is engaged in rendering professional advice or services to the reader. All matters regarding health require medical supervision. Women who are pregnant or nursing should ask their health-care practitioner prior to starting any of the programs discussed in this book. Pregnant and nursing women should not do the 90-day anti-candida program. The author and the publisher shall not be liable for and specifically disclaim any loss, injury, or damage allegedly arising from any information or suggestions in this book. The author and publisher are also not responsible for the reader's specific health or allergy needs that may require medical supervision, or for any adverse reactions to the recipes or products contained in this book. It is the reader's responsibility to ensure his or her own health and medical needs are met.

HarperCollins books may be purchased for educational, business, or sales promotional use. For information, please email the Special Markets Department at SPsales@harpercollins.com.

FIRST EDITION

Designed by Bonni Leon-Berman

Library of Congress Cataloging-in-Publication Data has been applied for.

ISBN 978-0-06-267125-7

18 19 20 21 22 LSC 10 9 8 7 6 5 4 3 2 1

To the late Dr. William G. Crook:
As promised, I carry on your mission
to help heal millions.

CONTENTS

FOREWORD

At every crossway on the road that leads to the future, each progressive spirit is opposed by a thousand men appointed to guard the past.

—Maurice Maeterlinck, Belgian Nobel laureate

Despite *Candida albicans*'s thirty-year history as a well-defined and well-described clinical entity, the concept that a diverse range of seemingly disparate symptoms could be attributed to systemic overgrowth of this yeast species remains foreign to most medical practitioners. The unfortunate consequence of this naïveté is that countless sufferers of this malady know nothing about the medical and lifestyle interventions that can pave the way to their recovery.

The relative obscurity of this disease in mainstream medicine is not the only problem. Many of the time-honored practices of today's health-care paradigm, including the excessive use of antibiotics and steroid medications—as well as the neglect of such simple practices as the use of probiotic beneficial bacteria—are actually setting the stage for the development of systemic candidiasis. As a result, those of us who deal with this health condition in the clinical setting are witnessing what now seems almost epidemic.

In her groundbreaking self-published book *The Candida Cure*, Ann Boroch offered readers a comprehensive understanding of this disease and its relevance to our health. Ann's firsthand personal experience, coupled with extensive and exhaustive research, resulted in a text that will surely stand as a fundamental resource in the emerging story of candida as the hidden cause of many illnesses.

Unfortunately, Ann passed away before she could see this updated and revised volume of her work published and distributed. But she did complete the revised manuscript before her death, and we know that she saw it as her mission to ensure that this information made it to those who are desperately in need of healing.

The Candida Cure deftly weaves together a compelling text describing the magnitude of the problem, its causes, and its cures, offering hope to those whose lives have been affected by this chronic condition. For it is hope that is drained from the countless undiagnosed and inappropriately treated candida patients who stumble helplessly from doctor to doctor. And it is hope restored that is the highest merit of this book.

That is Ann's legacy to us all.

David Perlmutter, MD, FACN, ABIHM

THE CANDIDA CURE

INTRODUCTION

When I was twenty-four years old, life as I knew it came to a screeching halt when my nervous system went completely haywire. For six to eight months I faced inexplicable daily episodes where I'd lose control over my motor skills, and my body would spasm and tremor uncontrollably. I experienced numbness and tingling in my limbs, muscle weakness, impaired sensory perception, bladder dysfunction, and nervous exhaustion. I wasn't able to talk, chew, or swallow in any normal way. I also had trouble formulating thoughts and accessing my memory.

After a neurological exam, an EEG to measure electrical activity in my brain, and evoked potential testing to determine how my nerves responded to certain stimuli, my internist announced his unsettling diagnosis. "Well, the great news is that you don't have cancer," he said. "The bad news is that you have multiple sclerosis." After that, everything became a blur as the words *incurable* and *deterioration* echoed through my head. Sick to my stomach, terrified and shocked, I looked at my poor mother, who was completely offended by the doctor's abrupt and insensitive manner. Together, we staggered out of the office.

When my doctor suggested chemo as a first step, everything inside me screamed that I needed to find an alternative route to conquering this so-called incurable disease. This was 1989, so there was no Google, and there wasn't much information out there about unconventional ways to deal with, much less recover from, MS. I had, however, faced candida issues when I was around eighteen years old, while battling mono, so I'd been initiated into the world of holistic diet, health, and candida overload to a certain extent. I knew that *Candida albicans* is a harmless yeast, a type of fungus that lives naturally in everyone—men, women, and kids alike. In a healthy body, candida lives symbiotically in a balanced environment in the gastrointestinal tract, on the mucous membranes, and on the skin. Unfortunately, however, this harmless yeast can overgrow and turn into an opportunistic pathogen.

I believed candida was the primary culprit in what was happening to me.

Research validated my suspicions. I learned that yeast/candida overgrowth and fungal toxins are a major factor in all autoimmune diseases—including, but certainly not limited to, MS. An autoimmune condition is one in which the immune system works overtime to defend itself against one or more rogue pathogens—so much so that it aggressively attacks the body's own cells. Think of it as friendly fire gone awry. To calm down my immune system and remove the burden that a candida overgrowth creates, I turned to Dr. C. Orian Truss and Dr. William G. Crook's landmark books on the topic, which drew profound correlations between autoimmune disease and yeast. I also dug into Judy Graham's *Multiple Sclerosis* for guidance. I put myself on a strict anti-candida diet, took an antifungal remedy and broader antimicrobial solution called Candida Cleanse by Rainbow Light, replaced fifteen silver amalgam fillings in my mouth (I nearly died in the process, as I'd temporarily become even more symptomatic after removing a quadrant of fillings), and used nutritional supplements to heal my immune system. I also worked through emotional and mental layers of fear-based patterns, because I truly believe that what you think about, you bring about, and that negative belief systems and patterns can affect cellular memory.

With time and tenacity, my body began to heal. The daily immune system attacks became less aggressive after six to eight months, and bladder and cognitive issues improved after the first year. Fatigue came and went. Numbness and tingling and impaired sensory perceptions lasted the longest. I'll be honest, it wasn't necessarily a smooth upward trajectory—central nervous system diseases rarely are. The central nervous system controls everything in the body, so it reacts to the external environment each day, along with having to tackle an existing condition. Stress and fear also play a big part in how candida affects the immune system and adrenals. The incredible news is that I found that most symptoms that seemed to be new or fleeting were just part of a healing crisis—and, knowing this, I could push through the discomfort with hope and optimism. As time went on, I became more confident about how to ride the waves and trust my body's ability to eventually right itself.

After four tumultuous years of struggling with MS, I finally triumphed over the disease at the age of twenty-eight. I put my debilitating condition into remission for good, and in the twenty-four years that have passed since then, I'm thrilled to say that I have enjoyed robust health and have not experienced any signs or symptoms of MS since.

Heal Candida, Heal Yourself

My journey made it feel clear that I now had a greater purpose—to help as many other people heal the way I did—and the best way I could think to do this was to write a book. Back in 2009, however, there wasn't a publisher around who was interested in putting out a book on candida. So once again, I took this on myself by self-publishing my protocol and diet plan for ridding the body of candida overgrowth. The book became an amazing best seller, and I received letters and e-mails from some of the nearly 70,000 readers who followed my protocol and experienced incredible results. Most had stumbled upon *The Candida Cure* by googling their symptoms and having a eureka! moment right there on the Amazon page. Far too many people were tired of feeling lousy and not getting answers, and desperate for advice. My book was just the antidote they needed.

Over the years, I've heard from countless readers and clients who put their autoimmune diseases into remission the way I did, but also from those who've found relief from seemingly random and vague symptoms such as overwhelming fatigue, bloating, acid reflux, eczema, weight gain, sinus infections, and depression—all by curing their candida overgrowth. And while there are plenty of through-lines, every candida picture looks a little different. Some sufferers will be taken down after an infection that doesn't go away, when several courses of antibiotics tip the scales. Others have a poor diet, experience high levels of stress, or may be on birth control for several years, and over time candida overgrowth becomes an issue. In all cases, however, clearing infection and inflammation allows the immune system to heal the body, removing whatever burden is taking its toll.

My book's success also showed me that those in need of helpful, healing information went beyond the "candida community"—the patients and practitioners who are aware of and believe in the pervasive negative effects of yeast overgrowth. And after being in private practice for twenty years as a nutritional consultant and naturopath, I can confidently tell you that the candida problem is pandemic—it's so much bigger than I could have ever imagined. Antibiotics, steroids, stress, sugar, heavy metals, alcohol, poor diet, and birth control pills pervade our lifestyles and health care, and all are underlying causes for overgrowth. The good news is that my program has helped thousands of clients with all types of conditions to resolve their allergies, autoimmune diseases, endocrine imbalances, gastrointestinal disorders, depression, anxiety, and more, and it can help you too.

I believe that most health conditions that are not congenital will benefit by resolving candida overgrowth, and while I wouldn't go so far as to say that candida is the cause of *every* disease out there, it is commonly a very big piece of the puzzle. When you have yeast overgrowth, it lays the groundwork for pathogens to flourish and opportunistic microbial infections to take hold. Viruses come out of dormancy, parasites make themselves at home, and bad bacteria proliferate. In the process of purging the body of harmful candida overgrowth with a thoughtful diet and antimicrobials, you remove various types of infection and inflammation from it. This either eliminates most if not all of the symptoms, provides a clearer picture of what remains out of balance in the body, or both. My candida program is such a success because it helps clean up the immune system and balances the gut microbiome, where most health conditions begin and candida problems are known to thrive.

Do You Have Candida Overgrowth?

If you've bought this book, you likely either suspect you have a candida issue or have been told by a practitioner that you do. Or maybe you've simply heard about candida and the mycobiome, and thought your symptoms lined up with that of an overgrowth. The following questionnaire, developed by William G. Crook, MD, is one that I like to use in my practice to assess whether candida overgrowth is contributing to a client's health problems. That being said, know too that it won't provide you with a black-and-white yes-or-no answer. That's because it's challenging to diagnose candida overgrowth—even in laboratory tests. This is one reason candida is often dismissed or downplayed within the diagnostic protocols of the traditional medical establishment.

The truth of the matter is, even if your score says that yeast-related health problems are "possibly present," it's likely that you have some degree of overgrowth that warrants attention. The test will also give you an idea of how certain medications and habits lead to yeast overgrowth. Frankly, I believe that everyone living in today's world can benefit from doing a 90-day program to heal the gut and remove toxins and inflammation from the body, as my candida program does. It will also give you more energy and mental clarity, improve your mood, and help you lose weight no matter where you fall on the candida spectrum.

To take the quiz below, you want to pay the most attention to your "yes" answers—each time you circle one in section A, you'll then circle the point score next to the question. When you've finished the section, total your score and then move on to sections B and C, and then total those scores at the end of each section. At the end of the questionnaire, add together your scores for all three sections to figure out your grand total.

Section A: Health History

Point Score

1. Have you taken any tetracyclines (Sumycin, Panmycin, Vibramycin, Minocin, and so on) or other antibiotics for acne for one month or longer? 50
2. Have you at any time in your life taken other broad-spectrum antibiotics for respiratory, urinary, or other infections for two months or longer, or for shorter periods four or more times in a one-year span? 50
3. Have you taken an antibiotic drug–even for one round? 6
4. Have you at any time in your life been bothered by persistent prostatitis, vaginitis, or other problems affecting your reproductive organs? 25

5. Have you been pregnant two or more times? 5

One time? 3

6. Have you taken birth control pills for more than two years? 15

For six months to two years? 8

7. Have you taken prednisone, Decadron, or other cortisone-type drugs by mouth or inhalation for more than two weeks? 15

For two weeks or less? 6

8. Does exposure to perfumes, insecticides, fabric-shop odors, or other chemicals provoke moderate to severe symptoms? 20

Mild symptoms? 5

9. Are your symptoms worse on damp, muggy days, or in moldy places? 20

10. Have you had athlete's foot, ringworm, "jock itch," or other chronic fungus infections of the skin or nails?

Have such infections been severe or persistent? 20

Mild to moderate? 10

11. Do you crave sugar? 10

12. Do you crave breads? 10

13. Do you crave alcoholic beverages? 10

14. Does tobacco smoke really bother you? 10

Total score, Section A ________

Section B: What Are Your Symptoms?

For each symptom you experience, enter the appropriate number in the point score column:

Occasional or mild = 3 points
Frequent and/or moderately severe = 6 points
Severe and/or disabling = 9 points

Total the score and record it at the end of this section.

	Point Score
1. Fatigue or lethargy	______
2. Feeling "drained"	______
3. Poor memory	______
4. Feeling "spacey" or "unreal"	______
5. Inability to make decisions	______
6. Numbness, burning, or tingling	______
7. Insomnia	______
8. Muscle aches	______
9. Muscle weakness or paralysis	______
10. Pain and/or swelling in joints	______
11. Abdominal pain	______
12. Constipation	______
13. Diarrhea	______
14. Bloating, belching, or intestinal gas	______
15. Troublesome vaginal burning, itching, or discharge	______

16. Prostatitis ________

17. Impotence ________

18. Loss of sexual desire or feeling ________

19. Endometriosis or infertility ________

20. Cramps and/or other menstrual irregularities ________

21. Premenstrual tension ________

22. Attacks of anxiety or crying ________

23. Cold hands or feet and/or chilliness ________

24. Shaking or irritability when hungry ________

Total score, Section B ________

Section C: Related Symptoms

Although the symptoms in this section occur commonly in patients with yeast-connected illness, they also occur commonly in patients who do *not* have candida. For each symptom you experience, enter the appropriate number in the point score column:

Occasional or mild = 3 points
Frequent and/or moderately severe = 6 points
Severe and/or disabling = 9 points

Total the score and record it at the end of this section.

Point Score

1. Drowsiness ________

2. Irritability or jitteriness ________

3. Lack of coordination ______
4. Inability to concentrate ______
5. Frequent mood swings ______
6. Headaches ______
7. Dizziness and/or loss of balance ______
8. Pressure above ears or feeling of head swelling ______
9. Tendency to bruise easily ______
10. Chronic rashes or itching ______
11. Psoriasis or recurrent hives ______
12. Indigestion or heartburn ______
13. Food sensitivities or intolerances ______
14. Mucus in stools ______
15. Rectal itching ______
16. Dry mouth or throat ______
17. Rash or blisters in mouth ______
18. Bad breath ______
19. Foot, hair, or body odor not relieved by washing ______
20. Nasal congestion or postnasal drip ______
21. Nasal itching ______
22. Sore throat ______
23. Laryngitis or loss of voice ______
24. Cough or recurrent bronchitis ______

25. Pain or tightness in chest ______
26. Wheezing or shortness of breath ______
27. Urinary frequency, urgency, or incontinence ______
28. Burning on urination ______
29. Erratic vision or spots in front of eyes ______
30. Burning or tearing of eyes ______
31. Recurrent infections or fluid in ears ______
32. Ear pain or deafness ______

Total score, Section C ______
Total score, Section B ______
Total score, Section A ______

Grand total score (Add totals from sections A, B, and C) ______

Your grand total score will help you and your practitioner decide if your health problems are yeast-connected. Note that scores for women will run higher than for men, because seven items apply exclusively to women, while only two apply exclusively to men.

RESULTS:

For Women:

If you scored 180 or more: Yeast-related health problems are almost certainly present.

If you scored 120 or more: Yeast-related health problems are probably present.

If you scored 60 or more: Yeast-related health problems are possibly present.

If you scored less than 60: It's unlikely that yeast is causing health problems.

For Men:

If you scored 140 or more: Yeast-related health problems are almost certainly present.

If you scored 90 or more: Yeast-related health problems are probably present.

If you scored 40 or more: Yeast-related health problems are possibly present.

If you scored less than 40: It's unlikely that yeast is causing health problems.

Adapted from William G. Crook, MD, *The Yeast Connection Handbook* (Jackson, TN: Professional Books, 2000).

How to Use This Book

It's been seven years since I originally published *The Candida Cure*, and a lot has changed. Enter this updated edition, which includes the latest science not only on candida but also on gut health and its relationship to what we call the mycobiome, aka the fungal community within our bodies. I will also share what I've come to learn about the self-healing mechanisms of our immune system, candida's relationship to small intestinal bacterial overgrowth (SIBO), optimal adrenal functioning, and the devastating effects of sugar and processed foods on the nervous system. All these factors play an essential role in bringing your body back to its healthiest state.

In the first half of the book, you will learn what candida is, why most health imbalances begin in the gastrointestinal tract, where candida wreaks the most havoc, and how your body's natural defense systems can be your best ally against candida and other causes of illness. In the second half, we will focus on using nutrition as a means of healing. What's more, I'll show you how to create your own 90-day program to achieve a vibrant level of health with the help of user-friendly charts and supplement protocols, a two-week sample menu plan, and delicious recipes. To completely beat candida, you need to implement both the anti-candida diet, along with an antifungal, and additional supplementation to support detoxification and restore optimal functioning of the body. I'll share reader and client success stories about those who've conquered sugar and carb addictions that fed their candida problems, plus their tips for overcoming the flu-like symptoms that can appear as you begin to detoxify your body and the candida dies off. Though these symptoms are normal and transitory, this virulent fungus puts up quite a fight!

My hope for you is that after a month, your symptoms will begin to subside, and by 90 days, you'll feel fantastic. My program is not about deprivation but about a lifestyle change that will help you not only regain health but also age with quality. And as blood sugar levels normalize and overgrowth is tackled, even your sugar and carb cravings will disappear. Don't worry—if you have a bad day and fall off the wagon, just get back on the next. You don't have to be a perfectionist, but you do have to commit to reap the benefits. Thousands have done my program, and so can you. I've designed every step to make swift and positive changes happen. Let's get started!

PART I

The Hidden Factor in Many Illnesses

1

The Candida Epidemic

Many of the illnesses and symptoms that plague men, women, and even children today—from fatigue, bloating, and weight gain to prostatitis, brain fog, arthritis, allergies, ear infections, and depression—can be traced back to a surprising factor: an overgrowth of yeast called *Candida albicans*. This fungus is meant to harmlessly and naturally live in our bodies, and when you're in good health, it exists symbiotically with other bacteria in the gastrointestinal tract, on the mucous membranes, and on your skin. But when your gut is out of balance, candida can overproduce—and the result turns an otherwise harmless microbe into an aggressive and opportunistic pathogen that systemically wreaks havoc throughout your body. Think of candida as the heat from your kitchen stove. Most of the time you appreciate it because it gives you exactly what you need—say, hot soup on a cold winter's night. But if you let it get out of hand, its flames will catch the drapes on fire.

Could Your Illness Be Caused by Candida?

Yeast overgrowth, which most practitioners refer to as candida or candidiasis, is a pandemic concern that affects millions of people around the world. More than 150 species of candida have been identified, with six being the most commonly found in humans. Conservatively speaking, one in three people suffer from yeast-related symptoms or conditions. It's always funny to me that in my practice, women seem to associate candida with vaginal yeast infections, and men relate the word *fungus* to an issue with their toenails. The truth is, both assumptions are sadly naive; candida can affect many other body parts than what are typically known.

In addition to the common, everyday concerns I mentioned earlier, candida has also been linked to arguably more serious and debilitating illnesses such as autoimmune diseases like multiple sclerosis, fibromyalgia, autism, and mental illness. In every case, however, Western medicine has failed to cite most of the pathogens that cause the body and immune system to go haywire, and I believe fungi are often the culprit—if not part of a larger microbial concern. This is why patients who see me for serious conditions that are often considered mystery illnesses or incurable diseases by doctors not only overcome them on my program but also find that other, seemingly minor and intermittent health annoyances disappear because they, too, were caused or fed by candida. These include sinus problems, tinnitus, upper respiratory infections, PMS, eczema, fatigue, brain fog, fibroids, acne, heartburn/gastroesophageal reflux disease (GERD), prostatitis, and anxiety. All can be part of a larger and more complicated fungal infection that is far too easy to shrug off, lather with creams, and dull with ibuprofen until it culminates in a larger and more unwieldy problem. Left unchecked, candida continues to multiply, and over time yeast, which is a single-celled organism, will change form to become a full-blown pathogenic fungus that is capable of causing disease.

When candida turns pathogenic and thus systemic, it shifts into a highly aggressive and invasive form called mycelial candida, sprouting whiskery food-seeking roots that extend themselves throughout your gut much like a plant's roots. Candida's roots then puncture the gut and firmly anchor themselves into the intestinal lining of your gastrointestinal tract, causing the intestinal barrier to become more permeable. This is one of the many causes of a condition called leaky gut syndrome—leaky gut, for short, which we'll discuss in more detail in chapter 2, "The Origin of Disease"—and it's exacerbated by an increasingly upset balance of microorganisms in your intestinal lining. When the wall that separates your gastrointestinal tract from your bloodstream becomes permeable, the fungus and its toxic by-products can seep through the intestinal lining into your body's circulating blood, where they do not belong.

The Mycobiome 101

So much about whether we sustain or disrupt good health is dependent on the body's microbiome, a term coined in 2001 by Nobel Prize–winning geneticist and microbiologist Joshua Lederberg to describe the approximately 100 trillion microorganisms or microbes that exist within the human body.[1] Your microbiome is composed of the bacteria, viruses, and single-celled microorganisms such as algae, protozoa, and fungi that reside in and on our bodies. All have a tremendous potential to impact our physiology. They contribute to metabolic functions, protect against pathogens, and support the immune system—and consequently, either directly or indirectly, they affect most of our body's functions. Without a doubt these organisms are essential to life-sustaining processes such as digestion, immunity, and the production and assimilation of vitamins.

The mycobiome, however, refers specifically to the fungal population in your body, within the microbiome—and if you've never heard of it, you're not alone. As researchers at the University of Pittsburgh School of Medicine point out, the mycobiome is an understudied ecosystem despite the fact that it plays a pivotal role in our health: "Diverse mycobiome patterns are associated with various diseases. By interfacing with other biomes, as well as with the host, the mycobiome probably contributes to the progression of fungus-associated diseases and plays an important role in health."[2]

Biome: A naturally occurring community of flora and fauna.
Microbiome: All your gut inhabitants.
Mycobiome: Just the fungi.
Biome host: You.

While research is being dedicated increasingly to the study of the mycobiome, this delicate ecosystem is still understudied in comparison to the microbiome—which I find a bit frustrating, because so many patients could potentially regain their health and vitality if it were more widely recognized, studied, and addressed clinically. Dr. Mahmoud Ghannoum, director of the Center for Medical Mycology at Case Western Reserve University in Cleveland, Ohio, echoed my concerns when he wrote, "The scientific community has not heeded our advice with regard to the fungal components of the microbiome. As of November 2015, only 269 of more than 6,000 Web of Science searches for the 'microbiome' even mention 'fungus,' and the scientific search engine returns only 55 papers pertaining to the 'mycobiome.'"[3] However, after twenty years of finding little or no scientific data on this topic, I am beginning to feel more optimistic; new research acknowledges the fungal mycobiome as "a critical player in health and disease."[4]

When the microbiome and mycobiome in your gut are out of balance, a condition otherwise known as dysbiosis, candida isn't the only organism that multiplies; populations of other microorganisms explode as well. Today, clinicians like me are witnessing especially marked increases in two manifestations of this imbalance: small intestinal bacterial overgrowth (SIBO) and *Helicobacter pylori*. Often, these proliferate in tandem with candida overgrowth, because of the gut's dysbiosis. SIBO and *H. pylori*, then, can open the door for candida, and vice versa. Low stomach acid can also promote SIBO and candida, and hydrogen produced by bacteria can be an energy source for *H. pylori*. And if antibiotics are given for SIBO and *H. pylori* treatment, even when they are necessary in some cases, this too will promote candida growth. Even so, candida is still ignored by most doctors. When a patient sees me for any of these infections, however, I like to use a broad-spectrum antimicrobial remedy that addresses all kinds of infections at once. It's important to be thorough here!

Let's take a closer look at these two treatable conditions, in case your candida has set the stage for them. SIBO is an illness in which bacteria typically found in the large intestine begin to multiply within the small intestine. This can happen due to a variety of reasons, including too-low gastric acid and motility disorders that don't allow waste to move through the GI tract due to a lack of water or fiber, too much sugar, a fistula, an impaired ileocecal valve, adhesions, gas, medications, structural abnormalities, or neurological and muscular conditions that slow down the transport of bacteria and food, which then sit in the intestine for too long. It can also be caused by immune system dysfunction. An increased incidence of SIBO has also been linked to increased use of medications for GI disorders known as proton pump inhibitors, like Nexium, Prevacid, and Prilosec. Symptoms of SIBO include gas, bloating, abdominal pain, nausea, constipation, and diarrhea—with less obvious signs that include an inability to absorb certain vitamins like B_{12}, chronically low ferritin levels (which signal low iron stores), acid reflux and/or laryngopharyngeal reflux (LPR, or "silent reflux"), and inadequate pancreatic enzymes. As for *H. pylori*, this is a bacterial infection that can cause ulcers in the stomach and small intestine for some, creating mild symptoms like bloating, belching, nausea, and abdominal discomfort, even though in others the bacteria can remain in the body an entire lifetime without causing harm. *H. pylori* enters your body through food, water, or saliva contaminated by an infected person, and once inside, it destroys the protective lining of your stomach and intestines. Your body's digestive acids can then cause ulcers.

Conditions Exacerbated by Fungal Overgrowth

Autoimmune Diseases

ALS (Lou Gehrig's disease)	Multiple sclerosis
Chronic fatigue syndrome	Muscular dystrophy
Fibromyalgia	Myasthenia gravis
HIV/AIDS	Rheumatoid arthritis
Hodgkin's disease	Sarcoidosis
Leukemia	Scleroderma
Lupus	

Blood System

Chronic infections	Thrombocytopenic purpura
Iron deficiency	

Cancer

Cardiovascular

Endocarditis	Pericarditis
Mitral valve prolapse	Valve problems

Digestive System

Anorexia nervosa	Food allergies
Bloating/gas	Gastritis
Carbohydrate/sugar cravings	Heartburn
Colitis	Intestinal pain
Constipation/diarrhea	Irritable bowel syndrome
Crohn's disease	Leaky gut
Dysbiosis	Malabsorption/maldigestion

Skin

- Acne
- Diaper rash
- Dry skin and itching
- Eczema
- Hair loss
- Hives
- Leprosy
- Liver spots
- Psoriasis

Respiratory System/Ears/Eyes/Mouth

- Asthma
- Bronchitis
- Dizziness
- Earaches
- Environmental allergies/chemical sensitivities
- Hay fever
- Oral thrush
- Sinusitis

Endocrine System

- Adrenal/thyroid failure
- Diabetes
- Hormonal imbalances
- Hypoglycemia
- Insomnia
- Over/underweight

Nervous System

- Alcoholism
- Anxiety
- Attention deficit disorder
- Autism
- Brain fog
- Depression
- Headaches
- Hyperactivity
- Hyperirritability
- Learning difficulties
- Manic-depressive disorder
- Memory loss
- Migraines
- Schizophrenia
- Suicidal tendencies

Urinary/Reproductive

- Cystitis
- Endometriosis
- Fibroids
- Impotence
- Loss of libido
- Menstrual irregularities
- PMS
- Prostatitis
- Sexually transmitted diseases
- Urethritis
- Yeast vaginal infections

Virus

- Epstein-Barr virus

Where Did All This Candida Come From?

So how can your yeast balance become so unwieldy and out of control? The real question is, in today's society, how can it *not*? Remember, yeast overgrowth often occurs as a direct result of microbial imbalances in the gut. So when the bacteria that make up its protective microbiome's terrain are wiped out, yeast flourishes and overproduces. This can happen due to the use of antibiotics, steroids, birth control pills, and estrogen replacement therapy, as well as the effects of heavy metals. Diets high in refined sugars and carbohydrates, dairy products, alcohol, and processed foods also create the ideal conditions in your digestive tract for yeast to thrive. Add in chronic stress—which elevates cortisol, a hormone produced by the adrenal glands, which are responsible for pumping out adrenaline under acute stress in our fight-or-flight response—and you have a recipe for disaster, as cortisol increases blood sugar. Candida doesn't care whether the increased sugar in your body is the result of eating a candy bar or another tough day at work; it will use the sugar as fuel to reproduce. And whether dysbiosis is a result of poor diet, stress, medications, or exposure to environmental toxins, once an imbalance occurs, the yeast will continue to multiply and progress into mild to severe health conditions.

I'd like to take a moment to focus on the overuse of antibiotics, since this is such an enormous factor in candida overgrowth, and one of the most common that I see in my practice. Antibiotics, as you likely know, are drugs that prevent and treat bacterial infections, such as strep throat, sexually transmitted diseases, acne, Lyme disease, pertussis (whooping cough), and food poisoning by *E. coli* or salmonella. Penicillin, the first antibiotic, was discovered in 1929; by the early 1940s, doctors across the country were quick to write a prescription for this new "miracle drug."

While it must be acknowledged that antibiotics are life-saving medications, with great benefits particularly in controlling epidemics related to food, infections, and airborne bacteria, the overuse of these powerful drugs can actually make us sick. For example, many of my clients have been prescribed antibiotics when they have a cold or the flu—even though, as I'd hope we all know by now, colds and flu are viral infections and not bacterial ones. Antibiotics are useless against viruses, yet many doctors prescribe them anyway. The Centers for Disease Control (CDC) has estimated that, of the nearly 154 million courses of antibiotics prescribed every year, 30 percent may be unnecessary.[5] The damage doesn't affect only your gut. This overprescribing has been linked to the rise of "superbugs"—pathogens that have adapted or mutated to resist antibiotic treatment, the most common being the MRSA (pronounced "mersa") staphylococcus bacteria, often found in hospitals. Without newer, more effective antibiotics, an increasing world population makes these pathogens particularly hard to kill.[6] This puts us all at risk of not being able to fight deadly infections when we need to.

When you take an antibiotic, the antibacterial medicine kills both good and bad bacteria in your gastrointestinal tract. Antibiotics do not affect *Candida albicans*, so without friendly gut bacteria like *Lactobacillus acidophilus* and *Bifidobacterium* to keep the *C. albicans* population under control, the candida multiplies; yes, probiotics can help mitigate this concern, but by no means are they a complete answer to a complicated problem. The depletion of your microbiome, then, can have a devastating impact on your mycobiome—and, thus, your health.

In fact, it only takes one early-life dose of antibiotics to start the fire. One! For example, if as a child you were given antibiotics for an ear infection or strep throat, this would be enough to trigger a rise in your yeast levels.[7] Over time, subsequent lifestyle factors such as poor diet or high stress levels would continue feeding the yeast until you became symptomatic of the next infection or condition. The vast majority of my clients have been prescribed several doses of antibiotics at some point. Some were rightly prescribed the treatment to help combat a life-threatening disease, but many others were prescribed the drug to treat substantially less dangerous conditions, like acne. A report in the *Journal of the American Academy of Dermatology* found that the average duration for antibacterial treatment for acne was 331.3 days, with more than a third of those patients on antibiotics for a year or longer.[8] The study's lead author suggested that if acne isn't controlled in six to eight weeks, alternative treatments should be initiated. In fact Jason, a client who suffered from persistent hay fever, told me at one point, "I was shocked when my wife made me check out your questionnaire for candida—because, well, I thought it was a woman's disease. But you say if somebody scores over 90, he's got it—and I scored 250. I took antibiotics for acne off and on all through high school—for years." Perhaps it's no surprise that the greatest incidence of candidiasis can be found in North America and the industrialized countries of Europe, where we see the highest incidence of antibiotic use, through both prescriptions and the consumption of animals treated with antibiotics. Antibiotics create conditions in the body that serve as a banquet for yeasts; and yeasts, in turn, serve as a banquet for viruses. When the delicate cohabitation of fungi, viruses, and bacteria is out of balance, viral infections can even create secondary bacterial infections. For example, the *viral* influenza can turn into *bacterial* pneumonia, which is, in turn, treated with more antibiotics, which creates more yeast, which attracts more viruses—and then you have a degenerative cycle that continues to perpetuate yeast growth.

The Vicious Cycle of Antibiotic Overuse

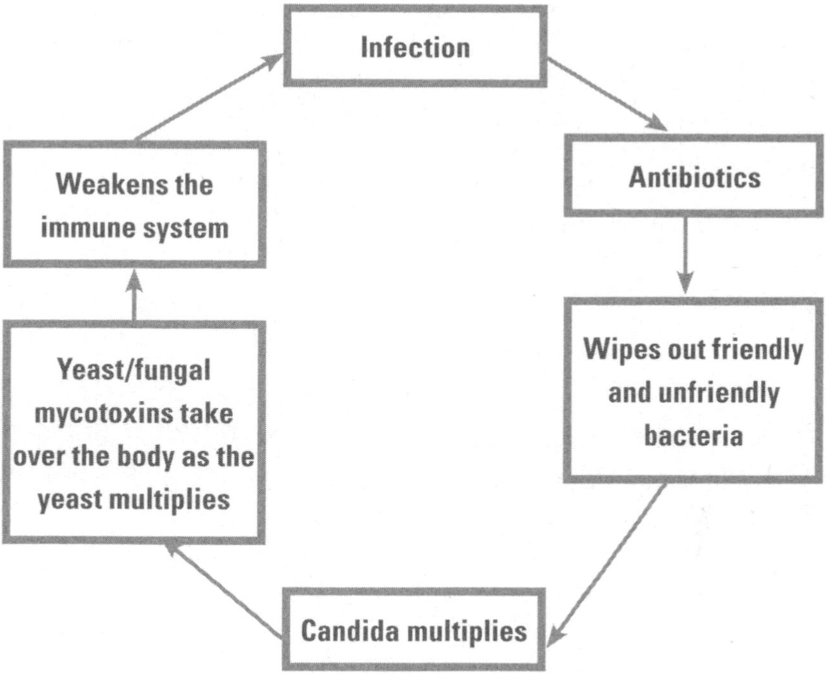

Reprinted courtesy of William G. Crook, MD, *The Yeast Connection Handbook* (Jackson, TN: Professional Books, 2000). Used with permission.

Finally, while few of us have escaped multiple prescriptions for antibiotics, I'm willing to bet that none of us have escaped ingesting antibiotics through our food sources. An estimated 70 percent of antibiotics manufactured today are fed to cows and chickens to prevent infection caused by the poor housing conditions of industrial farming. Unless you are always eating antibiotic- and hormone-free animal protein and dairy products—which means avoiding most restaurant meals, some dinner parties, and most packaged foods—you're "taking" more antibiotics than you realized, and thus have a higher likelihood of candida that's run amok.

Mycotoxins: Candida's Toxic By-Products

Once candida is in an overgrowth state, the body has to deal with not only an overabundance of yeast but also toxic fungal waste molecules called mycotoxins that are produced when yeast metabolizes glucose and other sugars through fermentation. The reason for the production of mycotoxins is not yet clearly understood, though we do know it's necessary for the growth or development of fungi. There are approximately seventy-nine different mycotoxins associated with *C. albicans*, all of which attack by weakening your immune system, causing inflammation in the body,[9] and destroying vital tissues and organs. These include acetaldehyde and gliotoxin, which I'll discuss more deeply in a bit, plus tyramine, canditoxin, polysaccharide proteins, histamine, and glycoprotein toxin.

Powerful mycotoxins can cause far-reaching breakdowns in your body. They're known to upset the communication of cell interactions. They can also disrupt RNA and DNA synthesis and damage and destroy neurons. They are carcinogenic and can induce ataxia, or a lack of coordination, and even convulsions. Since candida toxins commonly escape through the gut lining when it's become leaky, and enter the bloodstream, the hope is that the liver can then detoxify them. However, if the liver's detoxification ability is impaired due to inadequate nutrition and toxic overload, the liver can't do its work as a filter and these toxins will settle in other organs and tissues, such as the brain, nervous system, joints, and skin. Over time, other chronic diseases will then occur.

There are two major toxins produced by *C. albicans* that especially concern me, because of their significant impact on immune strength. The first, acetaldehyde, is the same by-product as that of alcohol metabolism and is six times more potent than ethanol; it also causes cell mutation. Clients with high levels of acetaldehyde from candida can even test positive on Breathalyzers! Normally, a healthy liver can convert acetaldehyde into a harmless substance. However, if there is an excess of acetaldehyde and the liver becomes oversaturated and can't keep up with demand, the toxin is released into the bloodstream, creating feelings of a hangover, brain fog, vertigo, and loss of equilibrium. And while the majority of acetaldehyde is processed in the liver, other tissues and organs can be involved and therefore affected, including the pancreas, kidneys, brain, and gastrointestinal tract.

Acetaldehyde has several permanent and more destructive effects, particularly with neurological implications. For one, it alters the structure of red blood cells, leading to a severe form of anemia and even cancer. Acetaldehyde destroys dendrites, threadlike segments of neurons (nerve cells) that pick up information from neighboring neurons and transmit it to the nerve cell body. It can alter neurotransmitters and normal brain function, bringing about lethargy, depression, impaired memory, and brain fog. Acetaldehyde also creates a chronic deficiency of thiamine, or vitamin B_1, which is critical for brain and nerve function and for the production of acetylcholine, one of the brain's major neurotransmitters, the chemical messengers that carry signals between neurons and other cells in the body. Moreover, thiamine deficiency is often correlated to cognitive symptoms such as emotional apathy, depression, fatigue, insomnia, confusion, and permanent memory loss. Acetaldehyde also depletes niacin, or vitamin B_3, which your cells need to burn fat and sugar for energy—and when your cells can't burn fat stores, you gain weight and feel lethargic. Niacin also plays an important role in the production of serotonin, a neurotransmitter that affects mood and sleep, as well as the production of a coenzyme that helps break down alcohol. Finally, acetaldehyde reduces certain enzymes in the body that help to produce energy in all cells, including brain cells.

Other signs of acetaldehyde damage include slow reflexes, heightened irritability, decreased mental energy, increased panic and anxiety, decreased sensory acuity, increased tendency to alcohol and sugar, decreased sex drive, and increased PMS and breast swelling/ tenderness.

Gliotoxin, our second mycotoxin of concern, deactivates important enzymes that move toxins through the body and causes DNA changes in the white blood cells, suppressing the immune system. Both of these consequences mean that your body is less able to detox efficiently, and the liver recirculates toxic metabolites. As fungus and mycotoxins continue to weaken your immune system, more infections arise, and you end up at the doctor's office again—being prescribed more antibiotics that perpetuate the vicious cycle.

Mycotoxins and the Mucous Membrane

One of the most remarkable characterizations of candida overgrowth is that it can factor into countless diseases. It doesn't discriminate against any body system—they're all up for grabs. This is because while *C. albicans*'s mycotoxins primarily target nerves and muscles, they can just as well attack any and every tissue or organ, including the skin, depending on certain factors such as your body's genetic predisposition and your dietary and lifestyle habits—and they all reach their destinations in the same way.

To better understand how candida can make certain parts of your body sick, think of your body as having two layers of protection that keep out foreign invaders, your outside skin and your "inside" skin—your mucous membranes. Yeast must pass through these to do its damage. Your mucous membranes begin in your nasal passages and run all the way down to your rectum, affecting the digestive, reproductive, and respiratory systems. This tissue is the same from top to bottom, and if it becomes inflamed or irritated, the membranes become more porous, allowing foreign invaders to enter the bloodstream. This can compromise organs and immune function. In the journal *Infection and Immunity*, authors Michael J. Kennedy and Paul A. Volz insist that "the passage of viable *Candida albicans* through the gastrointestinal (GI) mucosa into the bloodstream is believed to be an important mechanism leading to systemic candidiasis."[10]

Once an "invasion" takes place, *C. albicans* and its mycotoxins accumulate in the body, causing cellular disruption within the immune system and your organs and tissues. Mycotoxins so severely debilitate the body that, as Kennedy and Volz go on to say, "victims could become easy prey for far more serious diseases, [including] immune deficiency syndrome, multiple sclerosis, rheumatoid arthritis, colitis, [and] schizophrenia."[11] Then, on a personal level, your own genetic makeup includes risk factors for hereditary disease, your general state of health, and the culmination of diet and lifestyle patterns that determine which system or organs will be affected. So if you have a family history of mental illness, you'll be more prone to fungus affecting the brain. If you have a personal history of fibroids and endometriosis, yeast can affect your reproductive system. Sometimes an injury can make an organ, joint, or system susceptible to fungal damage. Candida is an opportunistic pathogen that way. It hits you where you're already most vulnerable.

When Candida Causes Endocrine Imbalances

One of the more common manifestations of candida overgrowth that I see occurs in the endocrine system, which consists of the hypothalamus, the pituitary, thyroid, thymus, and adrenal glands, the pancreas, and the ovaries or testes. This complex system of organs and glands is the source of the hormones necessary for a host of essential functions, including growth, metabolism, sexual development and function, hunger and satiety signals, and sleep and mood. It's also incredibly vulnerable to candida, for a number of biomedical reasons.

Researchers have long documented the relationship between specific hormones and candida; for example, a study conducted at the University of Des Moines, Iowa, concluded that excess estrogen accelerates the growth and survivability of candida.[12] Perhaps it's no surprise that women taking estrogen replacement therapy and oral contraceptives also experience higher incidences of candidiasis.[13] In addition, candidiasis can *mimic* endocrine imbalances and possibly compete for receptor sites that are targeted by endocrine gland excretion. And in hormone-related conditions where candida is not the primary cause, an anti-candida program can help to alleviate the symptoms of hypothyroidism, adrenal fatigue, PMS, and hypoglycemia. This is because the primary aggravators of these conditions are a poor diet that's heavy in refined carbohydrates and sugar, and unmanaged stress. The secondary aggravator is yeast overgrowth. As I've mentioned, every bodily system is affected by yeast, and when you clean out the yeast and tap into the body's natural ability to heal itself, you will notice improvements across these systems.

Candida and the Gut-Brain Connection

Since the late 1990s, an increasing number of scientists have referred to the gut as the "second brain." Of course, not because your intestines actually "think," but because of the enteric nervous system, the previously overlooked network of more than 100 million nerve cells lining the digestive tract. This network facilitates a two-way communication channel—the gut communicates with the brain, and the brain communicates with the gut. This chatter is responsible for everything from anxiety-induced digestion problems to excited "butterflies" in your stomach. I'm reminded of the intimate mind-gut connection whenever I see a client who suffers from GI disorders after having been treated with antidepressant medications such as serotonin reuptake inhibitors (SSRIs). Serotonin is the neurotransmitter necessary for maintaining mood balance and regulating sleep. Eighty to 90 percent of it is produced in your gut, and the rest is produced by your brain.

Researchers are discovering new and fascinating pathways for disease-related processes to progress from the gut to the brain. One of the more interesting is a direct route via the vagus nerve, which extends from the abdomen to the brainstem. A 2016 California Institute of Technology study found a conclusive link between gut microbes and the development of Parkinson's-like movement disorders in mice,[14] and subsequent research out of Sweden, published in *Neurology*, discovered that the disease appears to be triggered by a protein in the stomach that in fact spreads to the brain via the vagus nerve.[15] I have to wonder if candida travels in a similar way, and I believe we should devote the time, energy, and funding to studying exactly what mechanisms yeast might use to cross the blood-brain barrier, affect or send messages to the brain from the gut, or travel a different pathway altogether. After all, a team of scientists at the University of Madrid recently discovered fungal infection in the cerebrospinal fluid and brain tissue of patients with ALS, and in a separate study, the same team found fungi-infected areas in the brains of patients with Alzheimer's.[16] How did they get there? In a 2016 article in the alternative medicine journal *Townsend Letter*, David Steenblock, an osteopathic physician from San Clemente, California, has shown remarkable success with reversing ALS in patients—and has suggested a new pathway based on his patients' medical histories. He's come to believe that the disease may occur after repetitive neck injuries that introduce an opening, or break, between the blood and cerebrospinal fluid; this, he hypothesizes, allows toxins to enter the spinal cord and cause injury and death to motor neurons. What's more, he believes the toxic infection in question is usually a combination of yeast and bacteria—and he estimates that 90 to 95 percent of these cases begin in the gut.

When it comes to mental and emotional well-being, gut-based origins play a role here too. Emily Severance, a researcher at the Johns Hopkins University School of Medicine, further advanced the mind-gut connection when she discovered a link between a history of candida infections and higher rates of mental illness, including schizophrenia and bipolar disorder.[17] It makes perfect sense that when yeast attacks the gut, the brain is subsequently affected. Nevertheless, many physicians still assume that all mental and emotional imbalances have psychological causes, such as neuroses or psychoses, rather than brain-related causes. Some studies even point to an infectious catalyst for certain psychiatric illnesses. For instance, multiple studies have shown that the antibiotic minocycline is effective in treating schizophrenia-related symptoms.[18] While I'm no fan of excessive antibiotics, I do believe this demonstrates that what we once too easily tossed off as a "mental symptom" could actually come from a pathogen disrupting normal brain function and physiology.

Having anxiety, depression, or any other psychiatric manifestation of an illness can be debilitating, and it's important to understand that the cause may not be purely psychological but also physiological. The mind-gut connection means that what you put in your body—the food you eat and any medications you take—impacts your nervous system, as well as your mood, energy, vitality, and weight. Mycotoxins from fungus need to be considered when tackling these conditions. When this is a contributing factor, clearing fungal overgrowth from the system will help clear your mind and bring your body chemistry back into balance.

Congratulations! You Now Know More about Candida Than Most Doctors

By now, it probably seems more than a little obvious to you that your health issue is either being caused or at least fed by candida. So how can this fungus that has such a significant and widespread impact on your health receive so little airtime in the media, and often none at most doctors' offices?

Part of the issue is that the Western medical model doesn't support a holistic view of the body. We have specialists for every body part and system—and yet few doctors look at the body as a whole and investigate how these systems overlap. As we've discussed, your gut health is foundational for your overall health. And yet how many gastroenterologists are considering the ways in which your abdominal pain might be linked to stress? How many endocrinologists are assessing your digestive health? Western medicine is divided into specialties, and until we look at the body as a whole, we will never recognize the underlying conditions for disease.

My other concern is that most doctors tend to look at symptoms as problems to be treated, instead of urgent signals from the body that must be carefully decoded. Instead of investigating the reason behind a digestive issue like heartburn, they hand us a pill. Instead of simply sending us home with a prescription for plenty of rest and good nutrition when we have the flu, they hand us a prescription for antibiotics.

While there are some doctors who will treat intestinal and systemic candidiasis, few medical doctors recognize it as a general health condition. Some of my clients have even had the unfortunate experience of having their concerns dismissed by their physicians. I remember one client telling me that when she asked if her skin rash could be from candida, her doctor pulled out a coffee mug that read "My MD trumps your Google search." Often doctors only recognize and treat *C. albicans* overgrowth in cases of oral thrush, vaginal infections, hospital-acquired infections, or conditions associated with HIV/AIDS. This is because medical training teaches that candida is more of a problem with patients who have severely compromised immune systems.

I feel the lack and lag of science have kept the medical community in the dark about where the systemic origins of most diseases reside—in the microbiome and mycobiome. Medical textbooks don't offer detail about the critical importance of leaky gut and dysbiosis. Also, with antibiotics, hormone replacement drugs, birth control pills, and steroid drugs accounting for hundreds of billions of dollars in prescriptions written each year—in 2015 alone, pharmaceutical sales in the United States were reported to be nearly $374 billion[19]—our priorities may not be in the right place. Our medical system is very dogmatic, so I don't think we can expect anyone to admit that we've been deliberately overlooking or at least wrongly medicating so much disease anytime soon.

The good news is that with my book, you now hold the answer to candida-related illnesses in your very capable hands. You have the information to explain and validate your symptoms, plus the tools to significantly improve your health. Let's now move on to a more detailed look at how your digestive tract and immunity are involved in candida-related disease processes, so you can better understand exactly why you'll focus on these factors so heavily during parts 2 and 3 of this book—the diet, supplementation, and maintenance plans.

2

The Origin of Disease

Every organ and system in your body is closely connected; the function of one impacts the function of another. A constant stream of communication takes place within our bodies—a kind of automatic feedback loop—so if one organ becomes compromised, another will try to compensate. The digestive and immune systems are no exception, and in fact they are particularly interrelated; they rely on each other for support and good health, but this also means that if one isn't working efficiently, it puts more stress on the other. After all, roughly 70 to 80 percent of the immune system resides in gut-associated lymphoid tissue (GALT) located within the gastrointestinal tract.[1] Because the gut's impact on immunity is so great, no matter what health issues a client has, I always start them off with my foundational program of cleansing and rebalancing the digestive system. This allows the body to begin its healing process from a far-reaching position of strength.

The digestive and immune systems work together, then, to either sustain your health or contribute to health problems and disease. For our purposes, the candida ball starts rolling from the time you ingest potential insults like antibiotics or sugary foods, which then lead to poor absorption of nutrients and minerals. Next, it progresses to an imbalance of microbes in or on the body called dysbiosis, which contributes to leaky gut syndrome and elimination issues. Finally, your liver function becomes compromised and immunity is weakened. The end result is disease. The chart below illustrates this progression simply and clearly, but I'd like to explore each factor individually to give you a better sense of how all the pieces come together in your body.

Digestive Tract and Immunity

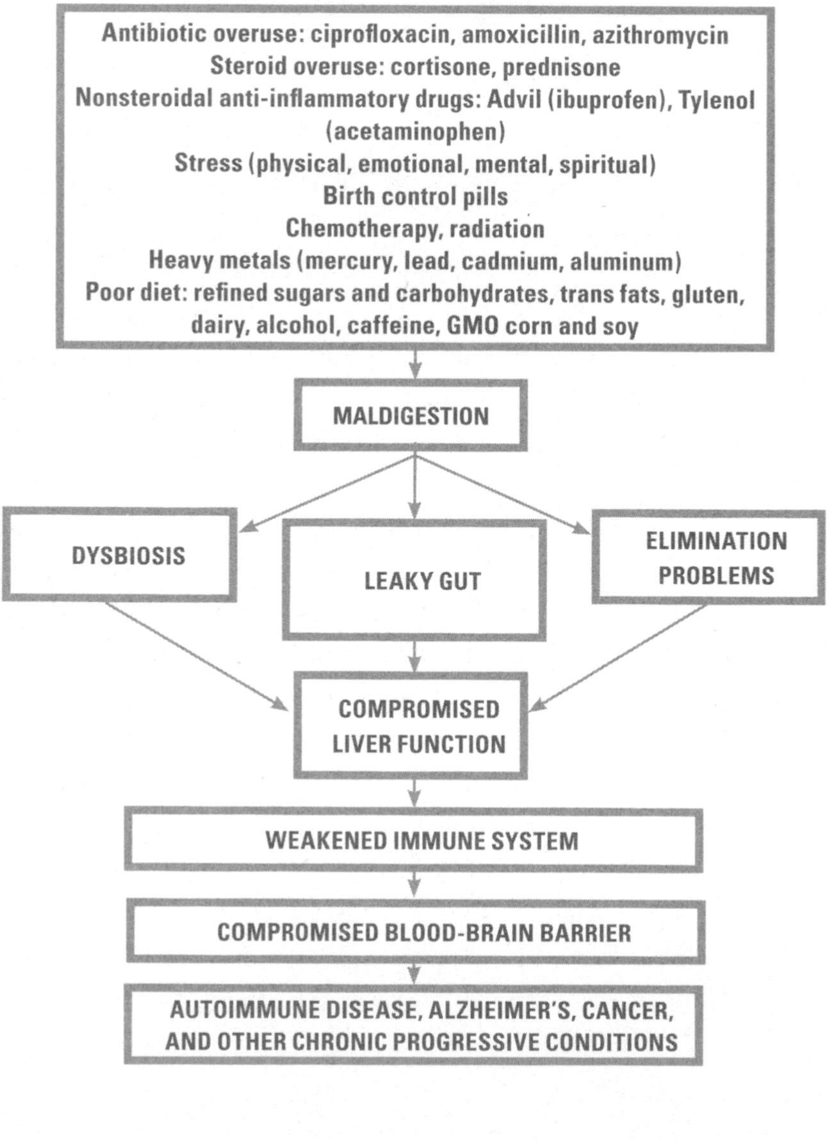

GI Symptoms: The Red Flag

Because of the gut's close relationship with your immune system, GI problems are always an important signal that something is going wrong systemically—and candida may be the very poison in the well. I'm always shocked when top medical specialists ignore diet and infection, including candida, as the source of serious gastrointestinal conditions, including ulcerative colitis, inflammatory bowel disease, and Crohn's disease, even after standard treatments fail to help many patients. It's hard to ignore the symptoms of digestive distress, and for good reason: the gut is the center of our health. More than 2,500 years ago, Hippocrates famously said, "All disease begins in the gut." But in recent decades those words seem to have been forgotten; most physicians view the gastrointestinal tract as a simple mechanism for processing food, absorbing nutrients, and filtering out waste. Fortunately, the National Institute of Health's Human Microbiome Project—a research initiative launched in 2008—has brought the focus back onto the digestive tract as the center of health and well-being.

Scientists tell us that there are ten times more bacterial cells living inside the GI tract—particularly the stomach and intestines—than there are human cells in the entire body. The small and large intestines alone have a combined length of twenty to twenty-five feet—the width of a tennis court—if you stretch them out. A balanced ecosystem in the GI tract has a ratio of 80 percent healthy microorganisms to 20 percent unhealthy ones. Poor nutrition can upset this ratio and create poor digestion, enzyme deficiencies, elimination problems, and intestinal dysbiosis. These problems are not isolated conditions that affect just the digestive system; they affect other systems of the body, especially the immune system.

Take Meghan, for instance. We first met when she wrote to thank me for the first edition of *The Candida Cure*. An otherwise healthy thirty-year-old professional, Meghan had been dealing with digestive problems her entire life:

> It seems like I always had an upset stomach, bloating, diarrhea, or constipation. It got worse when I was in college, and I had many embarrassing close calls sharing a bathroom with a roommate. Then in my junior year, I got very sick; I went down to 108 pounds and was put in the infirmary. Nobody knew what was wrong with me, so they pumped me full of antibiotics. Things did get better; but a few months later, all of my symptoms came back. My doctor told me I had IBS [irritable bowel syndrome], and by then I also was questioning my ability to digest dairy. The doctor prescribed Align probiotic supplements, and that led me to read a few books on digestive disorders. And I did get some relief cutting out high fat, fried foods, and dairy. But soon I hit a wall, and I was miserable again.

Meghan visited specialists and underwent all kinds of medical tests and procedures. She tried out every nutritional philosophy under the sun, including Paleo, blood type, low-fat, and low-FODMAP diets. Eventually she was diagnosed as gluten intolerant. She was also put on a protein pump inhibitor medication for acid reflux.

Many of the clients I see are at their wit's end when they land in my office, seeking relief from digestive issues that have been making their lives miserable. They've been to many doctors, and they've spent thousands of dollars on treatments, diets, and medications—all to no avail. While I'm frustrated that the medical system has failed them, I'm always elated that they found me so I can help connect the dots of their various symptoms. For Meghan, her GI distress was caused by a bad case of candidiasis. Following my protocol turned her health around.

Unlike Meghan, whose disparate GI symptoms managed to

stump all her physicians, my client Charlie, a forty-six-year-old website designer, had been suffering from what his doctors agreed was ulcerative colitis for fifteen years. Having a bona fide diagnosis, however, didn't get him any closer to relief, much less a cure.

"I can go months and be completely symptom free, or I can be housebound for months at a time," he told me. "And by housebound, I mean that I have to go to the bathroom ten or more times a day—with absolutely no advance notice. I can be sitting at my desk, and I have to jump up and run. Typically, it would start when I'd wake up, last through the morning, and then get worse again at night." Charlie told me that the disease had really limited his life. Because of his irritable bowel, he was forced to work from home. Even taking his son to school was a challenge, and when the disease was in a flare-up, even a simple task could be a real issue.

When Charlie was experiencing a flare-up, he'd often become depressed. He tried everything from supplements and probiotics to steroids and Vicodin, but nothing ever offered lasting relief. Eventually he found a specialist in irritable bowel syndrome and colitis who he thought would crack the case. Charlie said he was administered a series of food allergy tests, and in the end he was told he could eat anything but wheat, dairy, and almonds. But allergies weren't the issue. It was only in a follow-up visit that the doctor mentioned, as an aside, "You know, candida doesn't show up on tests." Luckily, those words led Charlie to my program.

Charlie's doctor made a good point: Because yeast can be evasive, hiding in tissues and organs, candida doesn't always show up on labs or in stool samples. Even if an individual is exhibiting all the symptoms, current tests won't show it. However, the more important takeaway from Charlie's story is that most of the time, doctors don't think to test for candida because they're looking for the wrong catalyst—but now you know better.

When Your Digestive System Breaks Down . . .

When your body becomes burdened from the antagonists we've discussed—antibiotic overuse, stress, a poor diet, and so on—the first sign of dysfunction that occurs in the gut is called maldigestion. Simply put, this is when the body is unable to properly break down food due to a lack of gastric juices (primarily hydrochloric acid) in the stomach, not chewing enough, pancreatic enzyme deficiencies, overeating, hiatal hernia, and stress. Drinking too much water or liquid with meals can also potentially interfere with the acid levels and bile needed by the stomach to properly digest your food. Another reason for maldigestion that's often missed but can cause distress is improper food combining. Not everyone has to follow this, but those with digestive and GI issues can find relief by following a few simple rules like eating proteins with vegetables and not starches, or eating starches with vegetables. Fruits are best eaten alone or with nuts. Fats do well with everything except fruit.

Enzyme deficiencies are another major contributor to maldigestion. Enzymes are proteins that accelerate the chemical reaction known as metabolism. While the body does manufacture its own enzymes, it must also obtain them from food. When foods are processed, refined, or cooked at temperatures above 118 degrees, their enzymes are destroyed. Raw or lightly steamed foods, on the other hand, are rich in enzymes. Signs of enzyme deficiency include bloating, constipation, hair loss, weak nails, fatigue, headaches, diarrhea, rashes, acne, and allergies. Some of the causes of this depletion include pasteurization and cooking at high temperatures that kill enzymes, heavy metals, pesticides and herbicides, and pancreatitis.

When the body is lacking in enzymes, the pancreas, which secretes digestive enzymes, takes on a greater load. The pancreas also produces insulin, the hormone that maintains blood sugar levels. Therefore, diets loaded with refined carbohydrates and sugar, plus cooked and processed foods, overwork the pancreas; this makes you more susceptible to yeast overgrowth because of increased blood sugar levels and undigested food particles.

When food goes undigested, the food particles can irritate the intestinal walls and cause increased permeability—this is to say, maldigestion is another cause of leaky gut syndrome. The undigested food particles can then cross the mucosal lining, where they enter the bloodstream. Your immune system reacts to these particles as foreign invaders and creates an antibody response by sending white blood cells to the rescue. However, this activity—this immune response—creates inflammation, and often results in allergic reactions and food sensitivities. In addition, the undigested food particles ferment in the gut, which fuels fungal overgrowth. Symptoms of maldigestion include belching, bloating, gas, abdominal pain, and heartburn.

. . . And You Can't Eliminate Your Elimination Issues

It shouldn't come as a surprise that when you can't digest your food properly, you either won't eliminate enough or you will eliminate too much—though with candida, constipation seems to be more prevalent than diarrhea. Physicians tend to underestimate the importance of elimination for overall health. Some of my clients have told me that their doctors advised them that daily bowel movements aren't necessary, and I couldn't disagree more. While it's true that everyone's digestion cycle is a little different—with some bodies taking twelve to twenty-four hours (those taking up to seventy-four hours are not healthy)—it is ideal to have at least one bowel movement a day.

Constipation can be caused by a host of factors, including adhesions, fibroids, and SIBO. A poor diet—one filled with processed grains and not enough fiber and water—is most often the culprit for poor elimination. Five years ago Dan, a thirty-year-old with a hectic work schedule, came to one of my nutrition courses because another client had told him the anti-candida diet could solve his problems with constipation and its secondary symptoms of brain fog, headaches, reactive hypoglycemia, and fatigue. He had a bowel movement only once every two to three days and was bloated and gassy. "I was pretty much raised on canned vegetables and snack cakes," he told me. After my 90-day program, Dan's constipation was gone for good. Not only did he feel better, but he also felt liberated from the junk food cravings that slowed him down. There was no question that candidiasis was his problem, because maldigestion and constipation created a fertile breeding ground for yeast.

Constipation is not only uncomfortable; it can be a serious health problem. When your bowels are backed up, a condition called autotoxicity can occur, which is when toxins aren't released from your body in a timely manner and become reabsorbed into the bloodstream. Constipation can make the pH level in the large intestine, which should otherwise be slightly acidic to neutral, more alkaline too. This creates a breeding environment for yeast, parasites, bacteria, and viruses to thrive and for candida to turn into a fungal form.

Dysbiosis, Leaky Gut, and a Stressed-Out Liver Create Disease

Maldigestion and intestinal dysbiosis work hand in hand when it comes to feeding disease. I like to define intestinal dysbiosis as an imbalance of several microorganisms in your gut flora—including yeast, bacteria, parasites, and viruses—that upsets the digestive system and interferes with nutrient absorption. Put another way, it's an imbalance of good to bad bacteria in the gut. When unhealthy microorganisms take over the gut—usually as a result of poor diet, excess alcohol, illness, heavy metals, medications, aging, and stress—your immune system becomes overly stressed to defend your body from these infections. Your gut then becomes a portal for infection, undigested proteins, and toxins to compromise the immune system—and it sets you up for inflammation and ultimately diagnoses that can include autoimmune disorders, diabetes, neurological conditions, breast cancer, and colorectal cancer. Candida overgrowth is one of the most common causes of intestinal dysbiosis.

There are many causes of leaky gut syndrome, as I've briefly mentioned earlier. These antagonists include microbes, mycotoxins, medications, alcohol, undigested food particles, toxins, chemicals, poor diet, chronic stress, and gluten. And when leaky gut is unaddressed over time, inevitable conditions like allergies, GI problems, fatigue, eczema, and autoimmune disease arise. Again, leaky gut syndrome occurs when the intestinal membrane becomes porous, which then allows undigested proteins, microbes, and toxins into the bloodstream. This process involves the wearing away of tight junctions found in the mucosal lining—think tiny little gateways that are meant to keep stuff inside your gut from sneaking out and into your blood. But when your intestines' mucosal lining becomes irritated, inflamed, and more permeable, those tight junctions get worn out. Candida, NSAIDs like aspirin and ibuprofen, poor diet, heavy metals, and the ingestion of certain foods like gluten all irritate the gut and loosen up these junctions, leaving behind microscopic holes that make the gut leaky.

A leaky gut makes your liver's job more difficult by forcing it to break down the undigested proteins and pathogens that have trickled into the blood via your now-permeable gut wall. The liver has many functions—it converts glucose to glycogen, produces cholesterol and bile, and stores vitamins such as A, D, K, and B_{12}—though detoxification is its primary job. But if the liver can't keep up with demand, excess toxins will be stored in the liver or recirculate in the body. When toxins recirculate via your bloodstream or the lymphatic system—which carries these dead cells, waste, toxins, and pathogens to the lymph nodes—they can get stored in tissues and organs, particularly fatty organs such as the brain, breasts, and hormonal glands. Essentially, these systems become overloaded and can't protect you as they normally would.

When pathogens and foreign organisms breach the gastrointestinal wall, immune cells inside the gut do their best to produce antibodies to neutralize these invaders and protect you from harm. This protective mechanism, carried out by white blood cells, is called the inflammatory response. It causes both a rise in body temperature and the production of these cells, all in the effort to isolate, destroy, and even expel the invasion. There are two types of inflammation: acute and chronic. For example, when you cut your finger, your immune system comes to the rescue and you experience the swelling, heat, pain, and redness of acute inflammation. Inflammation becomes chronic when your immune system continues to respond to a threat, as it does when it's triggered by a poor diet, allergens, and infections (fungal, bacterial, viral, or parasitical).[2] In fact, Tufts University molecular biologist Carol Kumamoto finds that "low-level inflammation promotes colonization of candida and this colonization, in turn, promotes further inflammation . . . which then delays healing."[3] Over time, microbes and toxins settle in organs and tissues such as the liver, brain, lungs, skin, and lymphatic system.

What's more, when it comes to neurological disease specifically, postdoctoral fellow Antoine Louveau and professor and researcher Jonathan Kipnis, both at the University of Virginia School of Medicine, have newly discovered a breakthrough understanding of the brain's immune response. They've found that the brain has its own system of lymphatic vessels—in a sense, *its own immune system*. Discovering a pathway for immune cells to exit the central nervous system raises the question of whether disruption to this route is involved in neurological disorders associated with immune dysfunction such as MS, meningitis, and Alzheimer's disease. As Kipnis said in a 2015 article in the online journal *NIH Research Matters*,[4] "We think these vessels may play a role in the pathogenesis of neurological conditions that have an immune component."

As you can see, imbalances in the digestive system impact the immune system in various complicated and cumulative ways—and disease is the inevitable and unfortunate consequence of this process. My anti-candida diet and antifungal regimen, however, can not only reduce inflammation but also restore your immune system and replenish your gut so your whole body returns to its optimal and most vibrant state.

ENCOURAGEMENT FROM DEB

My beginning symptoms were fatigue, poor memory, lack of focus, constipation, low motivation, and creaky knees.

I followed the anti-candida diet and recommendations religiously. Giving up coffee and sugar was hard at first, but after a few days, I felt better. As the weeks passed, people started commenting on how much better I looked. I knew the program was working!

Then the most amazing thing happened. About three months after starting the program, I noticed a normal elimination, my energy level shot up, and I could focus on my work. Because I felt so much better physically, my spirits soared. Now, after four months, I've lost fifteen pounds, and a routine blood test revealed the lowest cholesterol level in my adult life.

3

Using the Mind to Help Heal the Body

Like many ancient healing traditions, naturopathy was born from the belief that the body can heal itself when it has the right natural support and resources to do so. As a naturopath myself, I'm a proponent of related philosophies embraced by the French physiologist Claude Bernard, a man of great academic integrity and an early proponent of applying the scientific method to nineteenth-century medicine. Bernard's achievements were both impressive and vast—from pioneering the study of digestion to studying the role of the pancreas to the discovery of glycogen, a complex sugar substance stored in our liver and muscles. Bernard also believed our bodies possess a natural healing state that he called the *milieu intérieur*, "environment within." He believed that this habitat comes into balance when the physical, mental, emotional, social, and spiritual aspects of life are also in equilibrium. The state he described is what's commonly known as homeostasis.

In part 2 of this book, I'll provide you with every tool you need to bring your physical body back into balance. But right now I'd like to focus on the mental, emotional, social, and spiritual aspects of healing that are also important to reaching homeostasis. Given what I've learned from my own healing, plus the turnarounds in my clients, I'm certain that these factors will apply to you too.

Putting Your Mind in the Right Place

Naturopaths believe that the body has the inherent ability to restore, balance, and maintain good health—and that physical, mental, and spiritual balance is the means to achieve it. The connection between these core areas of wellness must be nourished and valued. This means that eating a healthy diet and managing your stress levels are just as crucial to your overall health as your mind-set, emotions, and spiritual life.

Mental and emotional strength are imperative to beating an illness like candidiasis. It helps to harness both to see your 90-day program through. Even so, you don't have to be perfect to heal your body; you simply need to be diligent and tenacious. Remember, there will be some days when you just don't want to eat what you're supposed to. Or you just don't have the energy to exercise. If that's the case, then don't. Get back on track the next day. You are developing a pattern of lifelong change; it's a marathon, not a sprint, and your healing will happen at a pace that feels right for you. In addition to a little mental fortitude, a positive outlook is important for success, plus your ability to sustain your enthusiasm for the program. Though your initial reaction to giving up certain foods, for instance, might be to feel overwhelmed or disgruntled, let's try not to view the program as a deprivation plan. Rather, take it in 30-day increments and consider reframing the challenge. Shift your perspective a bit. Instead of thinking about how upset you are about removing foods from your life, focus on how great removing inflammation and infection from your body will make you feel. Recognize that the program won't just help you get healthy now but help you age in a healthy way too.

Establishing a thoughtful, steady, and invested support system can also help you remain positive and proactive. You don't even need a big group of people to stand by you—having a spouse, partner, or friend who regularly checks in, asks how you're feeling, or even jumps on board with your protocol can be a real lifesaver. My client Andrew came to me with general symptoms of maldigestion, and after just two months together, he was completely symptom-free. One of his keys to success? "I could have *never* done this without my wife," he said. "She was perfectly healthy, but she immediately went on the diet with me for support. She threw out all her favorite snacks and sweets so I wouldn't be tempted." You can also find a tremendous amount of support in chat rooms and candida-related Facebook groups. Here you can share recipes, tips, information, and even emotional support from people all over the world going through the same challenges and with similar symptoms.

Throughout the program, it will help to watch out for negative and fear-based thinking. I understand that dealing with a body that feels out of control—teeming with random, seemingly inexplicable, and often debilitating symptoms—is downright scary. I've been there, and I have felt it in spades. But you may not realize the number of negative thoughts you have each day—whether they're about your health, job, relationships, what have you—and how much they impact your physical health. Most of my clients don't. An abundance of negative thoughts can lead to more stress in the body, which releases hormones like cortisol that slow down your healing. They can impact your gut and cause dysbiosis; heightened anxiety or anger leads to a queasy stomach, knots, and irritable-bowel-syndrome symptoms. Stress also shuts down digestive function, which fuels bacterial and yeast overgrowth and leads to dysbiosis. This, of course, impacts immune strength, as you learned in chapter 2. I've actually seen complex cases in which a nutritional program isn't enough to heal a client; mental and emotional roadblocks—say, a toxic relationship that brings daily stress that's harming the immune system—need to be removed. But when you find ways to neutralize fearful and negative thoughts, a smoother healing path unfolds.

Healing happens faster when there's a synergistic rhythm between the body and mind, but don't just take my word for it. Candace Pert, PhD, was an American neuroscientist and pharmacologist who discovered the opiate receptor, the cellular binding site for endorphins in the brain. She believed that receptor-active peptides, such as neuropeptides and immune system cytokines, were the agents that allowed for communication between the brain and body. Dr. Pert believed that the emotions we think about are stored in the body, at these receptors, and that expressing our emotions in a healthy way is key to integrating the mind and body. She also believed that negative emotions such as heartache, guilt, and anger can stay trapped in the body—and I couldn't agree more. In fact, in a 2004 study out of Southwestern University Medical Center in Dallas, Texas, scientists discovered that our experiences don't just live in our brains but are recorded at the cellular level in our bodies. They theorized that these cellular memories, so to speak, help spark illness and disease.

One technique that helps my clients release negative thought patterns is expressing themselves aloud. The first step, here, is to become aware of what thought or feeling is bothering you in that moment. Address it out loud by saying, "I am thinking . . ." or "I am feeling . . ."—and then just blurt it out. It's a great first step to accepting how you feel and dealing with it. For instance, if you're a sugarholic who's struggling to keep up with the program, and continually think about feeling tempted by and deprived of sugar, say aloud: "I am so angry that I can't have my chocolate. I just want a little piece every day. I accept that I'm feeling deprived and frustrated." Then take a breath and say, "This program isn't going to last forever. I can have chocolate again when I'm done. I have committed to doing at least thirty days, and I can do this." You can then take another deep breath, drink a glass of water, and have a snack that is on the program. When you express your feelings, acknowledge your reality, and then admit that you're okay with it in this way, you free yourself from—rather than feed into—a cycle of playing a negative loop in your head, which only ingrains it deeper. It helps to replace the frustrated thought or feeling with a positive one, plus a neutral action like taking a deep breath.

Most helpful of all, perhaps, may be to focus on how much better you feel as time goes on. Concentrate on the progress your body makes and how powerful it must be to heal itself with your support. Know that your body is doing everything it can to help you and is not fighting against your best interests.

Pay Attention to Your Spirit

When healing my own MS, I wasn't just focused on tackling candida and detoxifying the body; I made it a point to address all components of the mind-body-spirit equation—the last of which ended up carrying more of an influence than I initially thought it would. For me, it was critical that I felt connected to God, which gave me hope that I'd heal and helped me to trust and remain devoted to following my diet protocol.

I've come to believe that having faith and a spiritual connection to a higher power is essential to healing and remaining motivated to see a program through. One of the best ways I know to connect to your spiritual side is to explore meditation and yoga, especially since studies show that relieving stress, especially when you're ill, is actually easier when you feel connected to the spiritual aspects of life.[1] Research on meditation shows declines in self-reported measures of anxiety, stress, anger, and fear.[2] You can find great meditations on YouTube or apps such as Calm and Headspace. I also encourage visualizations like this one: at the end of every day, visualize putting all the "stuff" of your day—including problems and responsibilities—in a briefcase and closing it. Remind yourself that you can reopen the briefcase in the morning, but come bedtime, it's time to rest and restore the body. Other therapeutic rituals like chanting, going for a walk in nature, prayer, journaling, saying affirmations, or just making the time to be alone can help you connect to a deeper part of yourself and offer an opportunity to nourish a relationship with a higher power—God, Spirit, the universe, figures of faith, your higher self, or whatever it is that you believe in and that brings you peace and hope.

Another terrific way to tap into your spiritual side when healing is to listen to your intuition. I find that once clients are educated about candida and how to eliminate it, they become more in tune with how to listen to their body and even track the mechanics of how it's functioning. This is particularly key because it leads to self-reliance and knowing when to recognize symptoms and see the most targeted clinicians you can.

Most wonderful of all is that I've found that as your body heals from an illness like candida, your mind and soul move toward homeostasis as well. This is to say that when your healing is complete, your entire being is now revitalized too. Along the way, your thoughts become more positive, your mood improves, and you feel empowered to accomplish more than you ever thought you could, and hopeful about your new beginning.

ENCOURAGEMENT FROM CARLA

After many years of living with migraines, asthma, digestive problems, fatigue, and hormone imbalances—after seeing several doctors and having tests performed and never finding anything that worked to improve my health—I found this protocol.

It's been like a miracle and definitely a life-changing experience. For the first time in as long as I can remember, I feel great, have energy, and best of all, there's no more pain! It is such a wonderful feeling.

Yes, I had to make dietary—and life—changes; and yes, some of them are challenging to follow. But I only have to think of how great I feel to know it's so worth it. Since I've followed the program, my health, mood, and quality of life have never been better.

4

Candida Detox

In part 2 of this book, you'll begin my protocol to kill off as much fungus and excess yeast as you can to heal your candidiasis. Remember, you will never fully rid the body of yeast, nor do you want to—it is a natural part of a healthy, supportive internal ecosystem. So again, balance is what we're going for here. Achieving this goal requires a two-pronged strategy: (1), taking an antifungal supplement to kill the yeast overgrowth, and (2), modifying your diet to stop feeding the yeast in your body and keep it from overgrowing. You will do both at the same time, for the full 90 days, along with cleansing and support for your liver and gallbladder. In this chapter, I'll focus on how to use antifungal supplements to get rid of your overgrowth, detoxify your body from die-off, and troubleshoot the way die-off can make you feel. To me, detoxification is like hitting a reset button on your gut and immune systems to help your entire body function optimally again. It's worth the effort!

What Will My Detox Feel Like?

In my experience, I have found yeast and fungus to be evasive but stealthy. They hide out in organs and tissues, and therefore blood and stool tests don't yield conclusive results; this further allows them to thrive. Some clients even doubt they have a candida issue for this reason—that is, until they detox. Their die-off reactions make them acutely aware that their body's fighting a nasty battle on their behalf. You can feel it happening.

Starting a program that involves an antifungal protocol and food elimination can create what's called a Jarisch-Herxheimer reaction—a Herxheimer reaction, or Herx, for short—in your body. Here, you experience a host of physical symptoms that can last from a few days to a week or two—and for those with more severe conditions like diabetes or autoimmune or chronic respiratory diseases, it will go on for longer. As your body shifts into a self-healing mode, its cells release toxins and dead pathogens into the blood, and your elimination organs may not be able to get rid of them quickly enough. They then recirculate through the body, causing flu-like symptoms, abdominal distress, body aches, headaches, diarrhea, nausea, fatigue, fever, brain fog, and a worsening of your existing symptoms. Cleansing will make you feel worse before you feel better, but think of it this way: a Herxheimer reaction tells you that the program is working, and your body is doing its best to heal.

The beginning of your 90-day program is when your most intense die-off symptoms will take place. In your second and third month, you'll introduce a liver formula that may invite some mild die-off, but the bulk of discomfort happens in the beginning. If you were to stop the program for a while and go back to eating poorly, then resume the program, your die-off symptoms would likely recur—yet another incentive to stick with the plan once you've started! "Detox is nasty," says my longtime client Christi. "About two to three weeks after starting the protocol, I felt like I had the flu. I was extremely cold, nauseous, and had a splitting headache. Drinking huge amounts of water helped to flush the dying candida out of my body. But once it passed, I felt incredible! By then, I'd also lost eight pounds. My body started to really like what I was doing."

The most important part of helping your body cleanse itself of cellular debris and dying pathogens is to make sure that all your elimination pathways—your kidneys, circulatory system, bowels, lungs, liver, and skin—are supported and able to do their jobs. When it comes to healing from candida, it really is a group effort!

Cleansing Your Kidneys and Bloodstream

Your kidneys are two small, bean-shaped organs found at the base of your rib cage on the backside of your body. They filter around a hundred and fifty quarts of blood, which produces one to two quarts of urine, each day. Your kidneys work in conjunction with your bloodstream to remove waste from your body during the detox process.

To cleanse your blood and kidneys during your detox, I recommend drinking a lot of water. You'll aim to drink an ounce of water per two pounds of body weight, plus four cups of red clover tea, either hot or cold, to help purify your blood (see chapter 8, "Essential Supplements," for more information). So, for example, if you weigh 140 pounds, you would aim to drink about 80 ounces (six to seven 12-ounce bottles) of water each day, plus the tea. You may need to slowly work up to four cups of tea over time—it's okay to start out with just a cup or two a day. While red clover tea doesn't contain caffeine, it may initially keep you awake at night because it stimulates circulation, which can cause insomnia. If you're affected in this way—not everyone is—don't drink the tea past 5:00 p.m.

A NOTE ON RED CLOVER TEA

If you have any of the following health conditions, you should abstain from drinking red clover tea and instead drink one cup of hot water with fresh squeezed lemon first thing in the morning (on an empty stomach). You can also drink one to two cups of dandelion root tea or organic white tea—just keep in mind that the latter contains a small amount of caffeine.

DO NOT DRINK RED CLOVER TEA IF YOU:

- Have grass allergies
- Suffer from ulcers
- Have been diagnosed with acid reflux
- Are currently taking blood-thinning medicines.

If you are taking any kind of medication at all, please be sure to check with your doctor for potential interactions before starting to drink red clover tea.

If your die-off symptoms are so intense that you're feeling uncomfortable, you'll want to make detoxification easier on your bloodstream and kidneys. One way to do this is by cutting down the dose of your antifungals and red clover tea, and then slowly increase them again as you begin to feel better. There is no rush to reach full dosages; in fact, you might need to take one pill or drink one cup of tea for a full week before increasing a dose. You can also take molybdenum or sarsaparilla to help you tolerate detox. Chelated molybdenum binds with fungal endotoxins such as acetaldehyde, making you less symptomatic. Sarsaparilla pills or tincture also help with die-off because they bind with the endotoxins from bacteria and yeast. Ginger tea is great for nausea or a queasy or cramped stomach. If you have a headache that just won't lift, you can take an aspirin or ibuprofen to take the edge off. Remember, die-off symptoms are absolutely normal in the beginning of the program and will pass.

Before we move on, it's crucial to distinguish between an allergic and a die-off reaction. With an allergic reaction, you will experience hives, swelling of the throat, or intense itching on your body. If you have any of these symptoms, stop the antifungal, all supplements, and tea. Wait three days to let your body calm down, then reintroduce the antifungal, each supplement, and the tea one at a time. Note how your body responds for two days before adding another supplement or the tea. If you react again, discontinue that supplement or tea altogether.

Detoxing and Supporting Your Gallbladder and Liver

The gallbladder and liver work to filter and break down chemicals and toxins that need to be removed from the body via the kidneys and bowels. They, too, work in tandem during your cleansing process.

The gallbladder contains bile secreted from the liver. Bile—the emulsifying fluid stored in the gallbladder that helps break down fats and carry toxins from the liver, has antibacterial properties, and stimulates peristaltic action of the bowel—can become thick and sludgy after years of indulging in cheese, trans fats, and sugar. When bile gets sludgy, indigestion and constipation are common, and eventually the formation of gallstones can occur. You'll use a supplement during the first 30 days of your program to help decongest the sludge in the gallbladder; it contains herbs and vitamins such as dandelion root, milk thistle, taurine, lipase, and phosphatidylcholine. These herbs are cleansing to the gallbladder and liver, so there will be some die-off here too. That's why you'll want to work up to the antimicrobial gallbladder formula and red clover tea, which I explain further in part 2 of this book. Each one, in and of itself, can create die-off symptoms.

In the second and third months of your detox, you will focus on cleansing and supporting the liver, which serves more than five hundred functions, including assisting with metabolism, storing vitamins and minerals, and detoxifying hazardous compounds, as you've learned in previous chapters. One of your liver's many tasks is to recognize fat-soluble toxic substances such as heavy metals, pesticides, processed foods, alcohol, cigarettes, synthetic chemicals, medications, and the by-products of stress hormones and form them into water-soluble compounds that can be excreted via the bile and kidneys. To help support these liver pathways, I recommend taking a series of supplements during days 31 to 90 that include vitamins and herbs such as milk thistle, amino acids, B vitamins, vitamins E and C, artichoke, gotu kola, and panax ginseng. Details are included in part 2, as well.

Keep Your Bowels Moving

When you begin to detox, your bile will release toxins, and this can result in diarrhea and other changes in your elimination habits. You may even get constipated for a short time because your body is getting used to digesting new foods and going without others that were once staples in your diet.

As we've discussed, a daily bowel movement is essential to overall health—but two to three times a day is ideal, especially when you are detoxing. Even if you are consuming adequate amounts of fiber in fruits and vegetables and using the bathroom every day, I recommend added fiber in the form of one or two teaspoons of organic ground flaxseed daily, either in water, mixed with a hot cereal, or sprinkled on salads and vegetables. It not only helps you stay regular but also removes mucus, yeast, and by-products that have built up on your colon walls. If you're constipated, you will recirculate toxins and feel worse. Remedies for constipation are magnesium citrate, triphala, probiotics, or aloe ferox. Avoid supplements containing psyllium unless you have diarrhea, because it can create more gas and bloating. If you're still constipated after using flaxseed, add an herbal stimulant or magnesium citrate (for additional supplements that can help ease constipation, turn to chapter 8).

Purify Your Lungs and Breathe Easy

It may surprise you to learn that 75 percent of the toxins you eliminate will leave your body as you breathe, since your lungs filter out polluted air, foreign matter, and organisms that make their way in through the nose and mouth. When you inhale, oxygen enters the lungs and passes back out through tiny air sacs called the alveoli. From there, the oxygen travels to your blood through capillaries, where it's then carried to the heart to bring oxygen to your tissues, cells, and organs. When you exhale, the diaphragm moves up into the chest cavity. This forces air and carbon dioxide, a waste gas product, to be released from the blood and carried to the lungs for removal.

Many of us are what I call "lazy breathers," in that we tend to hold our breath throughout the day and breathe from our chests, versus through the engagement of our abdomen and chest as our bodies are meant to. It's important to be conscious of how you breathe, not only for the sake of this cleanse but because it greatly impacts your health long-term. My suggestion is to focus on deep breathing at intervals throughout the day. To do this, inhale starting from the belly up to the chest, and slowly to the count of 10. Hold your breath for 10 seconds. Exhale to the count of 10, starting from the chest and then down to the belly. Repeat ten times, three times a day. Not only do you bring more oxygen into the body this way, but you'll feel calmer and more focused. Deep breathing floods the body with more oxygen, which increases blood flow and clears carbon dioxide. More oxygen releases stress and anxiety by increasing neurochemicals that make you feel calmer and focused. It also alleviates muscle tension and ushers out toxins from the body. You can do this at work or at home, or go outside for a break and just breathe.

Cleansing the Lymphatic System and Skin

The lymphatic system is composed of lymph nodes, ducts, vessels, the thymus, the spleen, adenoids, and tonsils to move lymph fluid through the body. The lymph doesn't have the luxury of a muscle such as the heart to pump blood, so motion is needed by the joints and muscles to move lymph upward to be filtered by lymph nodes at the base of your neck. Sweating through the pores of your skin is another way that waste filters out of the body, and exercise is one of the best ways to move lymph through both motion and increased sweat. Brisk walking, swimming, isometric exercises, qigong, yoga, and even marching in place while you watch your favorite television show are all fine forms of exercise. Massage and deep breathing exercises also support your lymphatic system. Saunas and Epsom salt baths help with detox too, though those with more serious issues like autoimmune diseases, including MS, may not be able to tolerate the heat, which may do more harm than good.

Another simple practice that can help to increase your lymph circulation is dry skin brushing (you can buy a dry skin brush at your local health food store or online). This technique moves the lymph toward your nodes so they can filter pathogens and waste—a process called lymphatic drainage. Doing just a five-minute dry skin brushing can bring the same advantages for your immune system as a twenty-minute aerobic exercise; it also removes dead skin cells and promotes new cell growth. Before getting into the shower, brush your skin, starting with the bottom of your feet, with short gentle strokes upward toward your heart. Brush up your legs, up your back, and then over your shoulders and down to the upper part of your chest. Brush up your arms to the heart. Do not brush downward on your face, as the bristles can scratch. Brush for a total of three to five minutes, and be sure to brush gently. Lymph fluid sits right under the surface of the skin, so there's no need to do this in any vigorous way.

Another way to support this part of your detox is to use an ionic foot spa, a cylinder-shaped unit that you put into a footbath filled with water (see Resources, page 266). The ionic spa, through the electrolysis of water, produces positively and negatively charged ions or particles that are absorbed through the skin. This can improve cellular functioning and boost your energy so it's easier for cells to purge toxins. As with dry brushing, you don't need to overdo this technique to gain benefits. I suggest using the unit once every ten days.

Using Antifungal Supplements

For 90 days, I'd like you to take an antifungal supplement that's either herbal or pharmaceutical. Both herbal and prescription-strength antifungals are effective, though herbal antifungals are, in my opinion, safer, as the pharmaceutical antifungals can sometimes have unintended effects on the liver.

Herbal Antifungals

Herbal antifungals are readily available. You can find many of them at your local health food store, on Internet warehouse sites such as vitacost.com, or at a health practitioner's office. I have found the following brands to be the most effective for my clients (see Resources, page 266):

- Candida abX, from Quintessential Healing
- Candida Cleanse, from Rainbow Light
- Candida Support, from NOW Foods

What I love about these remedies is that they have antifungal properties that target yeast overgrowth, but also contain substances that are antiparasitic, antibacterial, and antiviral. You'll kill a lot of bugs with one treatment! Work up to the recommended dose slowly by starting with the smallest suggested amount, and before taking any antifungal remedy, make sure that your bowels are moving daily. If you're constipated before starting my program, take a week to first regulate your bowel movements so you're going to the bathroom every day.

If you have trouble finding any of the herbal products I listed above, look for yeast-eliminating items at your local health food store that have at least three to four of the following ingredients:

- Oregano oil
- Pau d'arco (lapacho)
- Caprylic acid
- Cellulose
- Black walnut
- Protease
- Garlic or allicin

Other effective ingredients include:

- Grapefruit seed extract
- Oregon grape root
- Olive leaf extract

- Phellodendron extract
- Coptis root
- Gentian root
- Berberine sulfate
- Ginger

What about Biofilms?

A lot of my clients ask if they need to take a specific enzyme supplement as part of my candida program to break down a component of candida called biofilms. A biofilm is a polysaccharide and protein matrix that acts as the fungus's protective shield; all microorganisms, including yeast, bacteria, and viruses, create them to hide from our immune system. Enzymes are typically suggested to break through candida biofilms, but I find that oil of oregano and protease, both of which are included in my formula Candida abX, are plenty effective. Also during my 90-day program, you'll be taking other products that have enzymes in them like hemicellase, cellulose, and protease, which break through the cell wall of candida, whereas not all antimicrobial herbs are effective at doing this. For over twenty years, clients have shown effective results by using everything from herbal antifungals to pharmaceutical antifungals, which we'll discuss next, without needing a specific biofilm product.

Pharmaceutical Antifungals

Prescription-strength antifungals include nystatin, Diflucan (fluconazole), Nizoral (ketoconazole), Sporonox (itraconazole), and Lamisil (terbinafine). These are good choices if your symptoms are chronic and severe, as with psoriasis, MS, fibromyalgia, lupus, and asthma; if you're in a wheelchair, however, nystatin and Diflucan may be too strong for your body to handle, since your circulation is compromised and toxins can't exit your body as efficiently. In this case, a probiotic, such as Flora 20-14 by Innate Response, is a safer choice. Also, because these antifungals require a prescription, I suggest talking to your physician about your condition to see if she is open to working with you (naturopaths in some states, like California, can prescribe pharmaceuticals too).

While herbal antifungals are effective, they are not as concentrated as pharmaceuticals, so you'll usually see results more quickly with a pharmaceutical. Be sure to discuss the side effects of these drugs with your doctor. If you go this route, I'd suggest using nystatin and/or Diflucan, as they've helped many of my clients. Nystatin is a concentrated extract of a soil-based organism that works by directly killing yeast. It comes in pill or liquid form. Do not take liquid nystatin; it contains sugar, which will only feed yeast. As the authors of *The Yeast Syndrome* write, "Nystatin is virtually nontoxic and nonsensitizing. All age groups . . . accept the drug without major side effects, even on prolonged administration."[1] Nystatin is not initially well absorbed into the bloodstream, but with prolonged use it does get there. The problem is that most doctors prescribe nystatin for less than six weeks, and you'll see results only if you use it for three months to a year. As for Diflucan (fluconazole), this is a synthetic antifungal drug that is effective against systemic candida overgrowth. It is much stronger than nystatin but also more toxic to the liver. If you use Diflucan or any other systemic antifungal (Nizoral, Sporonex, or Lamisil) for more than a week, be sure to have your doctor test and monitor your liver enzymes. If you have symptoms of severe depression and/or anxiety, a mental illness, or autoimmune disease, you can still use Diflucan to jump-start the eradication of the fungus. I suggest taking 150 mg Diflucan for a limited time only, three pills total, one pill every three days, and then switching to an herbal antifungal such as Candida abX or to nystatin. Diflucan primarily targets candida in the blood, whereas nystatin permeates the areas of the GI tract, where yeast overgrowth usually originates.

Adjusting Your Diet during a Detox

As you take antifungals, you'll also be on an anti-candida diet that I'll explain in more detail in part 2. Here, you'll eliminate all sugars, dairy products, refined carbohydrates, gluten, corn, and alcohol. You will also eliminate all yeast-containing and fermented products; these don't directly feed the yeast in your body but create an allergic or sensitivity response, so it's good to get rid of them to keep your body as clean as possible.

Killing off yeast overgrowth is hard work, but the detox process is proof that you're making great progress. Supporting your pathways of elimination and whole body with the right food is half the battle. Let's now take a more specific look at what it means to modify your diet to keep your yeast levels under control.

ENCOURAGEMENT FROM ALBERT

The Candida abX supplement is a wonderful product that really works! My husband has had celiac for ten years and strictly eats gluten-free. He also had stomach issues and problems digesting dairy and chicken, but this too has improved by following your program.

5

Starve the Yeast, Nourish Your Body

What you eat both on and off my 90-day plan is crucial to starving the yeast in your body and keeping future yeast from taking over. Because nutrition is always a sound foundation for good health of any kind, after three months I'll ask you to adjust your diet to fit a broader but still clean and low-candida menu. Everything you need to know about the specific foods you can and can't eat is detailed in part 2, but I'd like to talk here about what you'll generally keep in mind when following a healthy diet on my protocol now and for life.

I'm willing to bet that revamping your diet will transform your life in more ways than you realize. The best way to look at these changes is to realize that a healthy diet doesn't have to be about deprivation; it can be inspiring. Adopting a new way of eating is an opportunity to learn how to mindfully shop, cook, create new recipes, and share your lifestyle with your loved ones so that everyone benefits. It's also a misnomer that eating healthy won't taste good; it's just the opposite, actually. Your taste buds change when you eat well, and you actually crave more nourishing foods. I guarantee that educating yourself about what goes into a diet that fuels the energy, mobility, and strength to live your best life will urge you to make the best choices you can.

You Are What You Eat

Prior to treating myself for candida, for as long as I could remember, I'd been sick. As a child, I was riddled with colds, flus, and sinus and ear infections. Throughout my life, I was prescribed more than fifty-six courses or shots of antibiotics for various ailments. My diet until the age of eighteen consisted mainly of processed foods and sweets. I had a single, working mother, so I ate a lot of canned foods like Chef Boyardee, Kraft Macaroni and Cheese, and frozen TV dinners. I was addicted to sugar, and every day after school, I went to 7-Eleven to buy candy or treats like Ding Dongs, Twinkies, or Pop-Tarts. I easily devoured something sugary two to three times a day—and by the time I was thirteen years old, I had fifteen silver amalgam fillings to show for it.

When my body collapsed from the Epstein-Barr virus, also known as mononucleosis, at the age of eighteen, I believe this was my immune system's way of crying uncle. Usually three months of bed rest helps you heal, but it took me three times as long. After seeing eight different specialists, taking over thirty prescribed medications, and searching many months for answers on how to get myself well, I was still exhausted and suffering from brain fog, disorientation, constipation, shortness of breath, and dizziness. I had reactive hypoglycemia, dealt with random fevers, and was achy all over. I just didn't feel good in any way, shape, or form. Needless to say, this wasn't normal.

Serendipitously, as I was hunting for answers in a bookstore one day, Dr. William Crook's book *The Yeast Connection* caught my eye. I scanned through the pages and went right to his questionnaire, which I've included in the introduction of this book. I literally began to cry as I read down the list of symptoms—I had far too many of them, and it seemed stunningly clear that my EBV and candida were in cahoots.

I decided to take a leap of faith and try Dr. Crook's program, which consisted of following an anti-candida diet that included no refined sugars, dairy, white flour, or alcohol, and taking an antifungal remedy called Nilstat (nystatin). One long year later, I had regained my health. In that time, I learned an enormous amount about the role of diet in ridding the body of infection and inflammation. Unfortunately, I didn't realize how absolutely essential it is to stick to a maintenance plan after healing, and so I went back to my old habits of eating gluten, dairy, and sugar. I also didn't know that yeast overgrowth could roll into a debilitating autoimmune condition. Six years later, I was diagnosed with multiple sclerosis.

As I look back, the writing was always on the wall about the trajectory my body would take. I was a sugar addict until the age of eighteen, a type-A perfectionist with high periods of stress, and I was sick all the time with colds, ear problems, and sinus infections. I was continually put on antibiotics and steroids, which fuel candida. I had a mouthful of silver amalgam fillings, which added to my heavy metal load. Then EBV surfaced, which is common in those with MS. I'd also been put on several medications when my EBV wouldn't lift, since the doctors couldn't figure out what was wrong with me, and these invited more symptoms that fueled candida. All of these factors over time disrupted my microbiome and weakened my immune system until it simply stopped functioning as well as it should. I also believe that EBV doesn't really take down a body as hard as it did mine without candida overgrowth. It's hard to know which comes first—the yeast or the EBV—but I feel they go hand in hand.

As a naturopath who uses sound nutrition to help heal the body, I know firsthand the extent to which the food we put into our bodies isn't necessary only for survival but to create vitality and optimize the function of more than 300 trillion cells inside us. The digestion of food—as it breaks down into vitamins, minerals, fatty acids, and glycerol—has a complex chemistry, and what we eat can alter that chemistry either positively or negatively. Sadly, the average American diet consists of large amounts of trans fats, refined sugar, refined carbohydrates, corn, gluten, soy, caffeine, and alcohol—not to mention the chemicals and preservatives commonly found in processed foods. How can your cells thrive on food devoid of nutrition? They can't.

It's a mistake to think that eating the wrong food will not harm you. The equation is very simple: trash in equals trash out. A good diet is one of the most important means to prevent disease, as well as heal a diseased body. What you eat can either weaken or rebuild your immune system, speed up the aging process or slow it down. We can attribute some of the increase in health problems like allergies, diabetes, neurological disease, heart disease, mental illness, autoimmune diseases, and cancer to unhealthy diets.

The great news is that you have control over your food choices. Once you educate yourself about the problems you're facing, you can make the necessary modifications—and quickly notice improvements.

10 Foods That Upset Your Body's Balance

There are ten food categories that can feed unhealthy candida levels in your body and/or encourage poor health in general: refined sugar, trans fats, refined carbohydrates, dairy products, certain and excessive amounts of animal protein, excess caffeine and alcohol, food allergens, gluten, and artificial sweeteners and sugar alcohols.

1. Refined Sugar

Far too many packaged foods in your grocery store—from canned goods to breads to seemingly benign crackers—contain sugar, and as you know, candida thrives on it. In fact, researchers at the University of North Carolina found that a startling 68 percent of products in the US food supply contained some form of sugar. The United States is a nation addicted to sugar. In 1890 the average American ate ten pounds of sugar a year. Today, that figure is more than one hundred and fifty! Perhaps it shouldn't come as a surprise that a 2016 study published in the *Journal of Medical Mycology* compared the prevalence of candida in the oral cavities of diabetics and nondiabetics and found that the level was higher in diabetics.[1] Researchers concluded that there may be a positive correlation between glycemic control and candidal colonization.

Whether it's disguised as sucrose, fructose, dextrose, glucose, evaporated cane juice, high-fructose corn syrup, lactose, or maltose, refined sugar, which is usually extracted from sugarcane or sugar beets, is one of the most harmful substances you can consume. Sugar has absolutely no nutritional value on its own, and in fact it has a negative value in your body—it depletes the vitamins and minerals needed to sustain health. It wreaks havoc on the pancreas, which controls blood sugar levels, and weakens the immune system.

2. Trans Fats

Trans fats are obtained by infusing hydrogen into liquid vegetable oil, causing it to solidify. This is done for the sole purpose of preserving processed foods for a longer shelf life. They're also used as binders and fillers in pastries, breads, crackers, processed foods, microwave popcorn, chips, cookies, and margarines. In fact, the latest research shows that margarines made with trans fats—not butter—are the real cause of blocked arteries. They're difficult to metabolize, and so they collect in your body's fatty tissue. Trans-fatty acids are major contributors to heart disease, adverse effects on the brain and nervous system, diminished mental performance, increased risk of depression, cognitive decline, and even Alzheimer's disease.[2] Keep your eyes peeled while reading labels. Any food that lists "partially hydrogenated" or "hydrogenated" oil among its ingredients contains trans fats. Thankfully, you won't have to wonder about whether your food contains trans fats for much longer. The FDA has declared that all food companies must eliminate trans fats from their products by 2018. Of course, food containing them may still linger on grocery store shelves for a while, so it's important to read labels carefully.

3. Refined Carbohydrates

Refined carbohydrates such as white flour, white rice, and refined grains are commonly found in baked goods and desserts, breads, and crackers. I refer to refined carbohydrates as "glue and goo" because they coat the lining of your gastrointestinal tract in a sticky way and interfere with your gut's ability to absorb nutrients and eliminate waste. They also irritate the lining of your gastrointestinal tract, which contributes to leaky gut syndrome, and ultimately pave the way for inflammation and candida overgrowth.

If you read the ingredients label on a bag of flour, regardless of whether it's white or wheat, you will often find that it's been enriched with vitamins and minerals. This sounds better than it is. The truth is that when flour is bleached and refined, it loses important micronutrients, fiber in particular, which are still lacking after it's been enriched. Fiber is essential for proper elimination and for keeping blood cholesterol levels in a healthy range. Refined carbohydrates contribute to the alarming number of clients I see with constipation, irritable bowel syndrome, and imbalances in blood sugar levels because they convert rapidly to glucose, or sugar. Ingesting sugars on a continual basis can disrupt the pancreas and blood sugar function. This leads to both reactive hypoglycemia and diabetes. Reactive hypoglycemia and most cases of diabetes occur when your cells become resistant to insulin from the continual ingestion of refined carbs, soft drinks, candy, and other sugary foods.

4. Dairy Products

Cow's milk is one of the leading food allergens, and lactose—a sugar present in milk—feeds candida too. Consuming cow's milk—and the products that contain it such as ice cream, yogurt, and cheese—frequently causes sinus problems and gastrointestinal complaints. Asthma, headaches, joint and muscle pain, depression, lack of energy, and skin concerns are also attributed to dairy allergies, as is hyperactivity and irritability in children.

Having a milk allergy means that the body doesn't recognize the protein found in cow's milk, which it sees as a foreign invader, and defends itself by creating an allergic response. This autoimmune reaction generates inflammation. However, having a milk allergy is not the same as having lactose intolerance.

Lactose intolerance means that you lack the enzyme called lactase that breaks down lactose. In fact, researchers from the UK have estimated that 70 percent of people worldwide stop producing lactase sometime during childhood, increasing the likelihood of some degree of difficulty digesting milk sugar.[3] Lactaid milk, in which the lactose, or milk sugar, has been removed, was created for those who are lactose intolerant. However, removing lactose doesn't solve the problem for everyone who has a sensitivity to cow's milk. I prefer that you steer clear of both milk and lactose-free milk, since milk proteins can cause sensitivity and mucus in the body.

It is commonly believed that drinking milk is the best way to get calcium—after all, many doctors advise us to drink milk and to give our children milk. Women are especially targeted because we are more likely than men to develop osteoporosis as we age. Yet the fact is that milk is actually not a great source of calcium; only 30 percent of the calcium in eight ounces of milk is absorbed by the body. Pasteurization destroys the enzyme phosphatase. To maintain proper pH balance, the blood robs minerals, which are alkaline, from the body's biggest storehouse of minerals—the musculoskeletal system.

We are told that drinking milk is the best way to replenish calcium and other minerals needed for strong bones.

I *have* found that after my 90-day program, small amounts of unsalted organic butter and ghee are well tolerated. Small amounts of goat and sheep's milk and cheese can be okay too. For most people, both goat and bovine dairy products create inflammation, but there are exceptions. Whereas dairy products from cows are congesting to the body, goat and sheep products are less allergenic so easier to assimilate because of their molecular structure, which is similar to human milk. After the program, some clients like using Garden of Life's Goatein, a high-potency goat dairy powder that's predigested so it's easier to consume. Everyone is different, so pay attention to how you feel when it's time to test out foods after your three-month cleanse is done.

What's interesting is that humans are the only species that drinks milk from another species. And how do cows get their calcium? Not by drinking milk from another species but by eating grass, if they're humanely raised. I'm with the cows on this one. I believe it's better to get your calcium from organic plant sources than dairy products, contrary to what the media and most medical doctors would have us believe. Plant foods that are high in calcium—higher in some cases than cow's milk—include dark green leafy vegetables, sesame seeds, almonds, broccoli, and canned salmon and sardines. All of these also contain trace minerals that help calcium enter your bones.

5. Certain and Excessive Animal Proteins

Protein is essential to heal and repair the body, but if you eat animal protein, be selective about the source of your meat. When not raised organically, most pork, beef, chicken, and turkey contains antibiotics and hormones, which as we know can tip the scale in favor of yeast overgrowth. In addition, pork contains higher concentrations of parasites than other animal protein, and red meat is more acidic to your body chemistry, especially when cooked beyond medium-rare and when eaten with grains, beans, or starchy vegetables. Organically raised chicken and turkey are better choices. On the program, you are allowed to eat animal protein and fish.

Unfortunately, fish also contain toxins because our oceans are polluted with heavy metals and chemicals, so you want to make smart choices here. Shellfish are particularly high in contaminants, as they're bottom-feeders and absorb higher concentrations of chemicals and mercury. Wild-caught salmon, trout, halibut, sole, sardines, and cod are better choices, but even so, finding clean sources can be a challenge. Swordfish, mackerel, shark, tuna, and tilefish are highly contaminated with mercury and should be avoided.

6. Caffeine

Caffeine, whether in the form of coffee, soda, tea, or chocolate, raises blood sugar levels and is acidic. This is not the goal, since boosted blood sugar feeds yeast and a generally acidic environment contributes to inflammation. It stimulates the adrenal glands to release cortisol, as well. Small amounts of caffeine can be beneficial for the body, but overconsumption of caffeine can negatively affect the adrenals, which we depend on for optimal energy. The rise in cortisol also elevates blood sugar, which feeds candida.

If you do drink coffee after your 90-day program, be sure to buy organic beans. Nonorganic coffee is the most chemically treated food product in the world, and detectable levels of mold are often found in lower-quality beans. Decaffeinated coffee is even worse because of the additional chemical processing it undergoes to remove the caffeine, which is naturally occurring in the beans. If you purchase prepared coffee, I recommend switching your order to espresso, which is less acidic than filtered drip coffee. Drink no more than a cup of organic espresso a day to avoid upsetting your adrenal glands and blood sugar levels. After the cleanse, one cup in the morning is best for energy and focus; if you drink a second cup in the afternoon, you'll also be too tempted to reach for sugar.

Organic white tea, which has small amounts of caffeine, is an excellent alternative for coffee during and after your cleanse. Not only is it a blood cleanser, it will not disrupt your endocrine system the way coffee can.

7. Alcohol

All alcohol is a neurotoxin that goes directly into the bloodstream, creates an inflammatory response, and depletes vitamins and minerals in your body. However, while you're on my 90-day program, if there's a day that you decide to indulge in alcohol, it is better to drink a "dry spirit" like vodka because it is distilled and has less sugar compared to wine, beer, sake, or champagne, all of which are fermented and contain sugar that quickly feeds your yeast. After the program, I suggest testing the waters by having one or two drinks a week if you'd like. If you feel reactive, with a headache, GI upset, or hangover, consider drinking less or none at all. Dry spirits with club soda or a splash of cranberry are a better choice because they don't contain sugar.

8. Food Allergens

I find that food allergy tests come with many false positives. The reaction that most people are having is from acute food sensitivities that will dissipate once inflammation and infections are dealt with. Food allergy tests also flag foods that clients eat regularly as being a problem, but that is really not the case. Many of my first-time clients come in with their results showing that they can hardly eat anything, which leaves them feeling sad and deprived. I prefer to jump right into my 90-day program, which gets rid of dysbiosis and inflammation. If there are unresolved symptoms after 90 days, that would be the most accurate time to do a food allergy test.

What's the difference between food allergies and food sensitivities? A food allergy is more severe; it occurs when an immune system recognizes food as an invader and uses its antibodies to fight the allergen by releasing chemicals called histamines. Inflammation results, causing pain, rashes, and for some, severe reactions such as anaphylaxis. Food sensitivities are more benign, causing bloating, gas, and headaches.[4] The challenge with food sensitivities is to find out what is bothering your system because symptoms can be delayed and cumulative. Doing an anti-candida diet will eliminate most food sensitivities. There may be three or four foods that simply don't agree with you even after completing your program, but they'll be very easy to identify when you reintroduce them after the cleanse.

Food allergies and sensitivities arise when your gut is imbalanced and maldigestion occurs from consuming refined, depleted, and processed food. Large quantities of undigested food particles that irritate and pass through the GI tract's lining can cause an allergic reaction in the bloodstream. In addition to cow's milk, the most common food allergens are corn, soy, citrus fruits, chocolate, eggs, nightshade vegetables (eggplant, peppers, potatoes, tomatoes), and gluten. Allergies to certain fruits and nuts can also arise when your digestive system is out of balance. Before starting my program, you may have no clue about what's causing your symptoms because the reaction can be delayed for a day or two, and eating a food with multiple ingredients makes it hard to figure out what's causing the reaction. But when you heal your gut and strengthen your intestinal lining and immunity by eliminating your candida overgrowth, you'll find that you have fewer food sensitivities, or what was really bothering you becomes obvious because you'll add back foods one at a time.

Soy is one of the more common allergens I'm asked about, because it's been the topic of much debate recently. In America the market is flooded with genetically modified soy foods like processed tofu and soy protein powders, which research has shown may be harmful to your body. However, fermented soy products, such as miso and tempeh, are more digestible, and they are high in essential amino acids and B vitamins. Unfortunately, fermented soy products are not allowed on an anti-candida diet because they can aggravate candida.

A lot of people are allergic to soy and experience gas and bloating when they eat it. If you have this reaction, I recommend avoiding all soy products. There are also studies that say large amounts of soy protein can disrupt thyroid function. Because the jury is still out on whether soy is good or bad for you, I feel it is best to stay away from it.

In my experience, the best cure for food allergies and intolerances is abstinence. If you suffer from allergies or food sensitivities, eliminate trigger foods for at least one to three months to rid the body of inflammatory allergic reactions, which may include itchiness, hives, rapid heartbeat, fatigue, constipation, diarrhea, or canker sores. After a month, you can slowly begin to add trigger foods back into your diet. Your body will tell you if it likes them or not. If your body reacts, then you know to stay away from those foods or to eat them in moderation only. Variety is another way to avoid allergic and intolerance reactions. There are plenty of choices in each food group to ensure that you are not eating the same thing day after day.

9. Gluten

White flour, rye, most oats (due to cross-contamination), barley, spelt, kamut, triticale, and wheat contain gluten, a protein complex that is abrasive to the GI tract and can strip its villi, the hairlike projections attached to the intestinal walls that help to absorb nutrients and keep the gut clean of yeast and bacteria. In addition, wheat has been hybridized and is subject to a process known as gluten deamidation, in which it is converted to wheat isolates. These are used as binders and emulsifiers in foods, including meat products, sauces, soups, and some beverages. The isolates are more detrimental than gluten in native wheat and can cause inflammation in the body.

You can certainly have an allergy or sensitivity to gluten or soy, but because there's so much emerging data on gluten's relationship to candidiasis—and in the past ten years, I've seen more clients with gluten intolerance and celiac disease than ever before—I wanted to discuss this separately. A 2013 study published in the peer-reviewed medical journal *Lancet* finds that *Candida albicans* may act as a trigger in the onset of celiac disease in those who are genetically susceptible. There is a protein in *C. albicans* known as HWP1, whose structure is similar to that of gluten. When a candida infection is present in the gut, it can set off an immune system reaction to HWP1, which in turn causes an allergic reaction to gluten.[5] Several medical researchers have examined the link between gluten sensitivity and neurodegenerative conditions, as well. In a 2010 *Lancet Neurology* article titled "Gluten Sensitivity: From Gut to Brain," Dr. Marios Hadjivassiliou and his colleagues concluded, "Gluten sensitivity is a systemic autoimmune disease with diverse manifestations. This disorder is characterized by abnormal immunological responsiveness to ingested gluten in genetically susceptible individuals. Coeliac disease, or gluten-sensitive enteropathy, is only one aspect of a range of possible manifestations of gluten sensitivity. Although neurological manifestations in patients with established coeliac disease have been reported since 1966, it was not until thirty years later that, in some individuals, gluten sensitivity was shown to manifest solely with neurological dysfunction."[6] Interestingly, part of Hadjivassiliou's study revealed a segment of patients who had white matter lesions on the brain or spinal cord that were similar to those found in patients with multiple sclerosis.

If you want to know if you are gluten intolerant and/or are having autoimmune responses, you can contact Cyrex Laboratories (Cyrexlabs.com). Their Antibody Array 3 tests your transglutaminase reactivity, and their Antibody Array 4 lets you know if you have cross-reactivity to foods other than gluten. There is a strong relationship between transglutaminases testing positive and autoimmune responses. Those who test positive for transglutaminase and/or celiac disease must avoid gluten permanently. If you choose to get tested, I'd recommend waiting until after your 90-day program, when inflammation will be reduced, to allow for better accuracy.

10. Artificial Sweeteners and Sugar Alcohols

Artificial sweeteners such as aspartame, acesulfame potassium, saccharin, and sucralose are often promoted as an alternative to sugar for those who want to lose weight or eliminate sugar from their diets. But diet sodas and food products that contain these artificial sweeteners are very damaging to the body. The chemicals used to create these sweeteners, or to change the molecular structure of sugar to create them, are known carcinogens. Aspartame, a known neurotoxin, has been linked to neurological symptoms and conditions such as blurred vision, headaches, dizziness, memory loss, numbness, MS, ALS, and Parkinson's disease.

Sugar alcohols, such as erythritol, maltitol, mannitol, sorbitol, and xylitol, are rising in popularity because they are not as damaging to the body as artificial sweeteners. Ironically, these are neither sugars nor alcohols! They are carbohydrates with a chemical structure that partially resembles sugar and partially resembles alcohol, but they don't contain ethanol as do alcoholic beverages. They are incompletely absorbed and metabolized by the body and consequently contribute fewer calories than most sugars; however, because they are not fully absorbed, they can ferment in the intestines and cause bloating, gas, and diarrhea.

Of the sugar alcohols listed above, I prefer xylitol in small amounts because it is made by our bodies in the metabolism of carbohydrates, it raises oral pH to be more alkaline when ingested, and it is antimicrobial. Commercial xylitol is obtained from corn or the bark of birch trees. I prefer the latter to avoid products made with genetically modified corn. I suggest taking it only in small amounts (under one teaspoon, not daily) for two reasons. Xylitol is a carbohydrate, which means it will feed candida if used in large quantities, and although it is obtained from a natural source, it is chemically processed. Any artificial sweetener or sugar alcohol consumed in moderate to large quantities is toxic to the body.

10 Food Rules to Keep Candida at Bay

I know what you're thinking: *So what* should *I eat and drink?* A healthy diet, on and off my plan, looks like this: 60 percent organic vegetables; 20 percent organic animal protein; 15 percent gluten-free whole grains; and 5 percent organic fruits, nuts, seeds, beans/legumes (once or twice a week), and unrefined oils.

As you can tell, this is a very plant-based diet because a diet low in carbs keeps candida under control. Another major benefit is that fruits, vegetables, and plant foods are abundant in phytochemicals, which help prevent cancer and reverse disease. The most important vegetables to eat daily are dark green leafy vegetables—such as spinach, watercress, collard greens, mustard greens, turnip greens, dandelion greens, arugula, baby greens, bok choy, and kale—and sprouts. They are filled with vitamins and minerals, especially B_6 and magnesium, which are required for many metabolic processes. Cruciferous vegetables such as broccoli, Brussels sprouts, and cauliflower contain natural compounds that assist with healthy liver function. I do like the right animal proteins, because they contain all the amino acids required to keep your body functioning. Finally, raw nuts and seeds contain essential fatty acids needed for the cellular membrane around each cell.

1. Go Organic

The synthetic pesticides, fungicides, and herbicides used to treat conventionally grown food, including genetically modified foods, are carcinogenic—and they negatively affect the microbiome and gut lining, creating the underlying conditions for yeast overgrowth. While science hasn't fully disclosed all the negative effects that GMO foods may have on our bodies, it's best to avoid them. Genetically altered foods are filled with herbicides, which can damage our bodies. Studies link GMOs to kidney and liver damage, allergies, gastric disturbances, and cancer. Eighty percent of US corn and soy is genetically modified, and GMO corn is the base that we are using to feed all non-organic livestock and fish.

One of the best ways to avoid chemicals and get the best-quality nutrients possible is to support certified organic farmers and eat organic fruits, vegetables, meats, and dairy products. These foods are slightly more expensive, but your health is worth the investment. Quality outweighs convenience when it comes to healing your body. Be sure to wash all your fruits and vegetables with a little soap and water or a natural fruit-and-vegetable wash, which you can find in the health food store.

Animal Protein

When consuming organic animal protein, eat small amounts (two to four ounces per serving) at one time for optimal digestion, every day. One of the reasons I encourage animal protein is that it breaks down into amino acids when it's digested, and your body needs amino acids to regenerate and repair cells, tissues, and organs. Consuming meat also helps to keep blood sugar levels balanced. Eating animal protein fewer than three times a week can create deficiencies in your body such as fatigue, muscle mass loss, anemia, joint pain, and moodiness.

When it comes to choosing organic animal proteins, remember that lean options such as chicken, turkey, eggs, and fish are best. Some do well with red meat—lamb, buffalo, bison, and grass-fed beef are good choices. For those leaning toward vegetarianism, I suggest animal protein a minimum of three times a week. When choosing meat, as much as possible, make sure it is from free-range animals not given hormones and either grass-fed or given vegetarian and antibiotic- and GMO-free feed. Free-range chickens are not confined in small cages and may have a little more room to move around than chickens raised on factory farms. However, their conditions are not necessarily humane or sanitary, and they are often kept in crowded sheds or lots. Ideally, the best meat to eat is from pasture-raised animals, who are truly free to roam outdoors. Eggs are also a good source of protein and best prepared poached, soft-boiled, sunny-side up, or hard-boiled.

One thing to know about red meat is that it contains high concentrations of saturated fat that can increase inflammation, but is usually tolerable in small amounts. If you do eat it, choose meat from grass-fed animals, such as bison and lamb, and eat it only once a week. Listen to your body; if you're craving meat, it could mean you're iron deficient (blood type Os, particularly, crave more red meat). When preparing red meat, cook it rare to medium-rare, as this leaves some active enzymes to help you digest it. It's best to eat meat with vegetables rather than starches, beans, and grains to make it less acidic and easier to digest. If you are still not digesting the meat well, you can try taking a protein digestive enzyme that contains hydrochloric acid (HCl) and pepsin.

All fish contain some heavy metals, yet their biggest benefit, as a good source of omega-3 fatty acids, outweighs this. Wild-caught salmon, trout, halibut, cod, sole, and most other white fish are great in moderation.

Vegetables

Organic vegetables are loaded with phytochemicals, which your body needs to help it regenerate. Over 4,000 such compounds have been found in plants and some of the more common include:

- Beta-carotenoids, found in green and yellow vegetables, benefit the skin, bones, and immune system.
- Lycopene, abundant in tomatoes, red peppers, and pink grapefruit, is essential to heart health.
- Lutein, a deep yellow pigment found in leafy greens, broccoli, and Brussels sprouts, is related to eye and heart health.
- The anthocyanidins found in berries and onions contribute to the health of your heart and blood vessels.

Because vegetables have alkalinizing properties, they help reduce acidity in your body, which reduces inflammation. Ideally 60 percent of your daily diet should be comprised of vegetables. Green leafy vegetables are among the most nutrient-dense, and I recommend eating them every day. And since cooking destroys important enzymes that your body needs for digesting and assimilating foods, the more raw vegetables and fruits you eat, the more enzymes and nutrients your body will take in. However, if your digestion is out of balance, you might find that initially, for about one or two months, you'll feel best eating only steamed or cooked vegetables and then gradually increasing your raw food intake with each meal—taking digestive enzymes along with both.

Culinary herbs also contain valuable phytochemicals such as vitamins, minerals, and antioxidants, and are used to ease heartburn and headaches. Remember to include fresh herbs in your meals whenever possible.

Last, don't forget to incorporate sea vegetables, such as arame, kelp, dulse, nori, wakame, and sea cabbage, which are rich in minerals, including iodine. Most of us are lacking in iodine, which is essential for optimal thyroid function. Sea vegetables also bind with heavy metals and radioactive toxins and move them out of the body, making them a great choice when you are detoxing.

Primary Benefits of Common Culinary Herbs	
Cilantro	High in vitamin K, essential for bone and blood health, helping in the removal of heavy metals and blood clotting
Rosemary	Rich in antioxidants that fight Inflammation and fungus. High in vitamins A and C
Parsley	High in vitamins B_1, B_3, and C
Oregano	Antibacterial and antifungal properties
Thyme	Rich in antioxidants and contains antiseptic and antifungal characteristics
Basil	High in flavonoids, antioxidants, vitamins A and K, and calcium
Dill	High in calcium, niacin, and antioxidants
Mint	Used for maldigestion and headache
Tarragon	One of the highest in antioxidant value, often used as an appetite stimulant, also inhibits blood clotting; rich in B-complex vitamins
Marjoram	High levels of beta-carotenes and vitamin A, resulting in antibacterial and anti-inflammatory properties
Sage	Rich in antioxidants and B-complex vitamins, vitamins A and C, and calcium

Fruits

Seasonal organic fruits contain many beneficial vitamins and minerals that help the body function optimally, are full of antioxidants that prevent disease, and are loaded with fiber that supports a healthy GI tract. That said, fruits are also high in natural sugars, so I recommend eating them in moderation. When you do eat fruit, berries are a good choice. They are lower in sugar than most other fruits, and the skins contain beneficial antioxidants. Even after you complete the 90-day program, I recommend limiting your fruit intake to one or two servings per day. A single serving is a fruit about the size of a baseball or $^1/_2$ cup of chopped or cooked fruit. Sugar content recommendations vary, but I've compiled the following chart based upon several nutrition advocacy groups.

SUGAR CONTENT IN FRUITS

Low-Sugar Fruits

lemon and lime	fresh cranberries	kiwi
rhubarb	guava	avocado
apricot	raspberries	tomato

Low-to-Moderate-Sugar Fruits

blackberries	tangerine	cherries
strawberries	nectarine	peach
figs	papaya	blueberries
grapefruit	orange	grapes
cantaloupe	honeydew melon	

Moderate-to-High-Sugar Fruits

pineapple	apple	prunes, raisins, dates, and any dried fruit
pear	pomegranate	
watermelon	mango	

IF YOU'RE VEGETARIAN, LOAD UP ON NUTRIENTS

If you decide to become a vegetarian, or already are one, make sure you're getting adequate nutrition. Most of my strict vegetarian clients are relatively unhealthy because they're not compensating for the nutrients they are lacking—such as certain amino acids and B vitamins—by avoiding meat. I've also found that many vegetarians tend to eat a lot of grains, refined carbohydrates, and sugar, all of which deplete vitamins and minerals and feed candida. Personally, I find that eating some animal protein each week is the easiest way to keep your body chemistry in balance when it comes to protein requirements. But if you choose not to consume animal protein, I recommend taking a free-form amino acid blend and B_{12} supplement.

2. Incorporate Whole Grains and Pseudograins

Whole grains, which are the seeds of grasses, and pseudograins, the seeds of broadleaf plants, are complex carbohydrates that have not been bleached or stripped of their fiber. They include amaranth, barley, brown and wild rice, buckwheat, corn, kamut, millet, quinoa, gluten-free oats, rye, spelt, teff, triticale, and whole wheat. Grains contain important B vitamins, which support your nervous system. Some are needed in the brain to support nerve cells and help synthesize neurotransmitters. They are also a good source of fiber and help to keep your colon healthy. The problem is, we're a nation that loves sugars and carbohydrates, and we eat too much of this food group, whether it's bread, tortillas, rice, or bagels. We only need about 50 grams of carbohydrates a day, less if you want to lose weight. Examples of 50 grams daily are ½ cup blueberries (9 grams), ½ cup cooked quinoa (20 grams), ½ cup raw broccoli (2 grams), 1 medium Granny Smith apple (16 grams), and ¼ cup raw carrots (3 grams). And as you know, carbohydrates feed candida.

The Paleo camp has taught us that grains and pseudograins contain lectins and phytates, proteins or plant toxins that bind to vitamins and minerals, inhibiting absorption. Lectins and phytates can also irritate the intestinal lining, causing leaky gut and inflammation. Does this mean we need to avoid them altogether? My answer is that small amounts of gluten-free grains and pseudograins are acceptable. I have been successful over the years in helping many people get healthy and get rid of their candida overgrowth while allowing gluten-free grains in their diets. While there's no doubt been an uptick in the number of Americans suffering from gut problems, I don't believe that grains are the sole villain responsible for these issues.

It's good to know, too, that soaking grains makes them more digestible by eliminating most phytic acid and reducing lectins. Thirty minutes to an hour of soaking and rinsing is sufficient, though many prefer to soak grains overnight. If you don't have time to soak your grains, at least give them a quick rinse to remove dirt, mold, and contaminants. They will taste better that way too! This applies to grains and pseudograins such as millet, brown rice, quinoa, buckwheat, and teff. Quick-cooking oats don't need to be soaked.

During your 90-day program, I'd like you to eat gluten-free whole grains (except for corn, which contains mycotoxins, and white rice) in moderation. For those with more chronic conditions or who aren't seeing enough positive benefits on the program, you may want to avoid grains for a month and see if you feel better. After the 90 days are over, I recommend living gluten-free and corn-free as much as possible because gluten can be an intestinal irritant and corn is usually GMO, containing the mold aflatoxin and chemicals that can be carcinogenic.

3. Enjoy Your Good Fats

Fat is an important component of any healthy diet. Your organs are made of fat—in fact, your brain is at least 60 percent fat!—and your body needs fat to build cells and nourish them. Essential fatty acids include omega-3s, omega-6s, and omega-9s. Your body does not make omega-3 and omega-6 fatty acids on its own and produces a limited amount of omega-9s, so you must include them in your daily diet. These good-for-you fats help regulate hormones, blood pressure, heart rate, and nerve transmission as well as reduce inflammation and pain.

Foods high in omega-3 essential fatty acids include deep-sea fish, dark leafy greens, coconut, flax, fish oil, hempseed oil, krill oil, olive oil, raw nuts and seeds, and avocados. Unsalted organic butter contains small amounts of omega-3s as well as vitamins A and D. Even if you consume these foods, you still need to take an omega-3 supplement because you won't obtain enough through your diet. Omega-6 essential fatty acids are found in eggs, grass-fed meat, raw nuts and seeds, and safflower, sunflower, and hemp oils. The best source of omega-9 fatty acids is olive oil, but they can also be found in almonds, avocados, and sesame oil.

Saturated fats from foods such as eggs, coconut meat and oil, butter, ghee (clarified butter), and grass-fed meat are beneficial in small quantities. These foods contain important vitamins and minerals, but you should eat them in moderation because large quantities can make the body acidic, which promotes inflammation.

4. Eat Beans and Legumes in Moderation

Beans and legumes are high in protein but also high in starch, which converts to sugar in the body that can feed candida. Legumes are also high in lectins, carbohydrate-binding proteins that can irritate the gut lining and lead to leaky gut. Because of this, I recommend eating small portions of beans and legumes only once or twice a week while on the diet or skipping them completely for the first two months of your anti-candida diet, particularly for those with an autoimmune disease. The two exceptions to this rule are adzuki and mung beans, which are higher in protein than other beans—it's okay to eat slightly larger portions of these. I suggest preparing beans with one or more of the following herbs and spices for optimal digestion and taste: cumin, clove, caraway, dill, fennel, sage, thyme, onion, oregano, ginger, garlic, rosemary, tarragon, and turmeric.

As I mentioned earlier, I recommend against eating soy beans and soy products, since so much of the soy in the United States is genetically modified and processed. The only soy that is permissible on the anti-candida diet is Bragg Liquid Aminos, an unfermented, non-GMO soy sauce.

Because phytic acid, which is the phosphorus store in plants, binds to nutrients, especially minerals, you're not able to absorb them. Soaking organic beans/legumes overnight and cooking the soaked beans in fresh water makes them more digestible by eliminating most of the phytic acid and thus avoiding flatulence. Some people with autoimmune conditions or chronic conditions will do best avoiding beans/legumes for three months to reduce inflammation. If you feel bloated, gassy, tired, or achy after eating beans/legumes, stay off them for one to three months after the diet ends and retest.

5. Choose Sweeteners Wisely

While you need to avoid sugar on the 90-day program, there are some sweeteners that do not feed candida and can be used in moderation: chicory root, luo han guo (monk fruit) extract, stevia, and xylitol. Even though xylitol is a carbohydrate, it is metabolized slowly and therefore does not increase sugar levels rapidly. Just make sure the brand you buy sources their xylitol from birch bark instead of corn. And while coconut sugar is popular for its lower glycemic index, it will still feed candida; it's best to wait to slowly reintroduce this after 90 days.

When your candida levels are back in balance after completing the program, you might be tempted to indulge in your old familiar sweeteners. Be careful, as sugar brings back candida with a vengeance. Most of my clients tell me they eventually lose their sweet tooth completely, and only eat sweets on rare occasions. If you really do need something sweet, raw, unfiltered honey and coconut nectar in small quantities (once or twice a month) are better choices than evaporated cane juice or agave. Raw honey contains amino acids, enzymes, vitamins, and minerals that are beneficial to your body. Coconut nectar has a low glycemic index.

6. Save Fermented Foods for After the Program

This one might seem a little counterintuitive because fermented foods are said to be great for the gut, but when you're balancing candida, they can initially aggravate overgrowth and present as an allergy response. These include sauerkraut, kefir, cultured vegetables, kimchi, kombucha, tempeh, yogurt, and nutritional or brewer's yeast—and I suggest staying off them during the program and then waiting three months to a year to introduce them to see if they agree with you. After all, not all fermented foods are made cleanly. Some have vinegars and pasteurized milk that cause candida flares. And then there's kombucha, which is made with wild bacteria and yeast and has small amounts of alcohol that can irritate candida. During and after the program, the exception to my no-fermented rule is raw unfiltered apple cider vinegar, which balances pH levels and helps rid the body of candida.

7. Consider Food Combining

Proper food combining involves eating either protein with vegetables or grains with vegetables but avoiding mixing protein with grains at the same meal. Doing this can benefit those with digestive problems. Others find that having a little protein along with grains at each meal, whether from an animal or a plant source, keeps both their blood sugar and energy levels more stable. The answer lies in listening to your body. If you're hypoglycemic, meaning that you have low blood sugar, start off your morning with protein and work your complex carbohydrates into your lunch or dinner meals. Most people who struggle with reactive hypoglycemia—low blood sugar after a meal high in carbohydrates and sugars—do best eating three meals a day plus a snack mid-morning and -afternoon, as this keeps their metabolism and energy levels balanced. If you are prone to excessive weight loss, however, eat only the three meals a day and avoid snacking in order to slow down your metabolism.

8. Drink Your Water

Many of my clients only drink between two to four glasses of water a day without my prodding, which is nowhere near enough to sustain a healthy body. As the eminent researcher Fereydoon Batmanghelidj, MD, states, "Dehydration is the number one stressor of the human body—or *any* living matter."[7]

Your body is 80 percent water. How can you keep it running smoothly when you drink fewer than eight cups of water a day? You can't. When you do, your "plumbing" gets backed up—your lymphatic system becomes sluggish, your kidneys become overstressed, your colon becomes constipated, and your liver and gallbladder become congested. Autotoxicity occurs as you reabsorb the toxins your body is unable to eliminate. These conditions set the stage for GI problems and autoimmune diseases.

And no, soda, coffee, iced tea, and fruit juices are not substitutes for water. These beverages do not hydrate the body and its organs in the same way that water does. Dr. Batmanghelidj explains that the brain is 85 percent water: "Next to oxygen, water is the most essential material for the efficient working of the brain. Water is a primary nutrient for all brain functions and transmission of information."[8] This means that your body needs adequate water if you want to stay sharp and focused. If you notice that your urine is dark in color, this indicates that you are dehydrated. Don't let yourself get to the point of feeling thirsty either. Drinking more water can eliminate a number of symptoms, including headaches and pain in the body.

As we discussed in chapter 4, "Candida Detox," you can easily calculate the ideal amount of water you need to drink: one ounce for every two pounds of your body weight. So if you weigh 150 pounds, you need to drink 75 ounces (a little over nine 8-ounce glasses) of water daily. Or to make this easier, just drink 6 ounces—a little less than one cup—every waking hour until you go to sleep.

Distilled water is a good water choice for hydration because the distillation process removes harmful chemicals and minerals (some controversial such as fluoride), which makes it almost pure water versus tap and bottled waters. This is terrific for cleansing toxins out of the body, but the downside is that it leaches essential minerals. If you drink distilled water, make sure to take your vitamin and mineral supplements daily. Sparkling mineral water in small amounts is acceptable as a soda replacement. Look for brands from Europe, which contain higher amounts of natural minerals and less added carbonation.

The best way to ensure that you're getting purified water is to buy your own filtration system (see Resources, page 266). I don't recommend most bottled waters because manufacturers are not regulated, and you don't really know what you're getting. Also, the chemicals from plastic bottles are endocrine disruptors (there are one or two water companies that deliver in glass bottles). If you do buy bottled water, look for a brand that states on the bottle how the water has been processed, such as through reverse osmosis. If this information is on the label, you have some assurance of the water's purity.

Believe it or not, herbal teas do count as water; but because they are also diuretics, make sure to put minerals back in your body by taking your daily multivitamin-mineral supplement. Among the many therapeutically beneficial teas are red clover, white tea (it has small amounts of caffeine and is an excellent blood cleanser), pau d'arco, rosemary, dandelion root, green tea (caffeinated or decaffeinated), chamomile, hibiscus, and mint. Green tea has also been found to have beneficial detox properties and epigenetic consequences.

Another great hydrator for the body is fresh coconut water, but it should only be drunk after exercising once you have completed your

90-day program, as the average-size can contains fourteen grams of sugar. You can also obtain small amounts of water from eating fresh organic fruits and vegetables.

9. Take Up Juicing

Juicing is a great way to nourish your body. Fresh vegetable juice immediately fills your bloodstream with live enzymes, vitamins, and minerals. Juicing is also alkalinizing to your body because it leaches out acidic waste products. Your digestive system doesn't have to work hard to absorb vitamins and minerals from juice, since the fiber is missing, which makes it an easier way to load up on vegetables on a daily basis. When you're juicing, be sure not to include large amounts of sweet vegetables or fruit; without the fiber, the juice is absorbed quickly and causes a rapid spike in blood sugar. If you want to eat a high-sugar fruit, eat the fruit itself or use it in a smoothie, where the fiber is beneficial and will temper blood sugar spikes.

Juicing correctly is important when you are using it as part of a health program. First, don't make more than eight ounces of fresh juice at one time. Drinking sixteen or thirty-two ounces of carrot juice at one time can do more harm than good, because vegetable juice can contain a lot of sugar. Below is a list of low-sugar vegetables that are great for juicing.

LOW-SUGAR VEGETABLES GOOD FOR JUICING		
celery	kale	broccoli
parsley	collard greens	cabbage
cilantro	mint	endive
cucumber	Brussels sprouts	asparagus
fennel	string beans	
spinach	red, yellow, and green peppers	

Second, drink juice on an empty stomach, either an hour before or two to three hours after a meal. Since the juice acts as a cleanser for your bloodstream, do not drink it with a heavy meal.

Third, drink your juice as soon as you make it. Many vitamins and minerals become oxidized within thirty minutes of being exposed to air.

Fourth, drink your juice slowly. Swish it around in your mouth to mix it with saliva, which releases digestive enzymes from your mouth, and then swallow.

There are many books on juicing that you can use to find recipes you like; see page 196 for the juice recipe I recommend most. When it comes to buying a juicer for your home, I recommend the Breville juicer, which can be bought online on Amazon or in many local department stores. The Vitamix food processor is a wonderful way to make soup, but it is different from juicing. A Vitamix retains the fiber, which your digestive system then has to break down, whereas juicing discards the fiber, allowing the nutrients in the juice to go directly into the bloodstream. Fiber is important to move stool through the digestive tract, normalize bowel movements, lower cholesterol levels, and balance blood sugar levels.

10. Be Sure to Nutritionally Supplement

In today's world, a good diet alone cannot keep your body healthy—and as you now understand, a healthy and well-nourished body is the very opposite of what yeast needs to thrive. If you want to experience good health and a balanced microbiome as you age, supplementation is essential, and you will find all the supplements you need to maintain great health both during and after the program in part 2 of this book. Because modern agricultural practices have depleted our soil, we must eat five times the amount of vegetables our grandparents ate to obtain the same nutrient value. Our bodies must also cope with more environmental toxicity from pesticides, herbicides, heavy metals, and synthetic chemicals than ever before. On top of that, increased stress levels have weakened our bodies, making supplementation necessary to offset the imbalance.

Now that you've seen how important it is to get rid of candida through a rigorous diet and supplement plan, it's time to officially begin the 90-day program. Are you ready? Remember, any lasting change takes time and dedication, but you're already well on your way to a candida-free body and revitalized life.

ENCOURAGEMENT FROM DAN

I was pretty much raised on canned vegetables and Little Debbie cakes. I'd never heard of quinoa, let alone been able to find it in the grocery. Now that I've learned what and how to eat, the thought of something like pizza grosses me out. All I can think of is all that cheese and dough! I still follow the diet about 70 percent of the time, and I have no more constipation issues at all.

PART II

Beat Candida in 90 Days

6

The Candida Cure

Your Path to Good Health Is Easier Than You Think

Now that you have a sense of the widespread effects of yeast overgrowth—and the foods and lifestyle choices that fuel that growth—you're probably ready to take action. The most important cornerstone of my anti-candida plan is nutrition, and in the pages that follow I offer a 90-day plan that will both nourish you and eliminate candida overgrowth. In a short amount of time, you will recapture your energy and vitality. For most people, it only takes a month to experience positive changes that will encourage you to maintain new, healthy habits.

I know that the prospect of changing your diet can be a challenge at first. Many of my clients are initially reluctant to give up their favorite foods. One in particular—Irina—comes to mind. Even after she was diagnosed with painful rheumatoid arthritis, she balked at the idea of abstaining from sugar. But after she stuck to the plan and experienced its benefits firsthand, she was hooked. Irina offered this encouragement for beginners: "After two weeks on the food protocol, I could sense a difference in my mental state. The depression eased and I started to feel like myself again. After three months, I saw enough clues and changes to absolutely know that I was healing. I relaxed because I was finally in control—and then, suddenly before I knew it, I was symptom-free."

The lists in this chapter offer an easy, at-a-glance reference for identifying which foods nourish the body and do not promote the growth of yeast, and which foods I suggest you avoid because they *do* promote yeast overgrowth. Be aware, however, that everyone's body chemistry is different. Some people have sensitivities or allergies to certain foods on the "Foods to Eat" list, so be mindful of your body's response to new or different foods, and take note of any experience of negative side effects. Symptoms such as fatigue, itchiness, rapid heart rate, gas, burping, bloating, constipation, diarrhea, and headaches are signs that you need to stay away from a particular food.

You will experience the quickest results within 90 days by adhering to the lists as closely as possible. For those of you who feel you are not able to jump right into the diet, I have included at the end of this chapter a slow-start plan that will allow you to eliminate offending foods gradually and move into the anti-candida diet with ease. Your progress, however, will be a little slower, adding about another five weeks to the program.

I have also included in this chapter two weeks' worth of sample menus so you can see that this diet is entirely doable and even enjoyable. You will discover that there are plenty of delicious meals you can easily create using nutritious foods. In chapter 7, "Delicious Recipes to Beat Candida," you will find recipes for main dishes, side dishes, sauces, desserts, snacks, and beverages as well as a list of the food brands I recommend.

Be easy on yourself as you begin to incorporate these changes into your life; you can't and won't be 100 percent perfect all the time, and that's okay. My client Lori—an executive working in a high-stress industry—describes herself as a perfectionist. She came to see me after having been diagnosed with lupus and found that this eating plan changed her life. Her advice for those new to the plan? "Focus on getting rid of the biggest offender in your diet. Build up from there."

I couldn't agree more. Once you've successfully eliminated the food that's giving you the most trouble and feels the hardest to sacrifice, the other changes to your diet will come easily.

Controlling Cravings

My number one rule—for everything, but especially when you're making a change to your wellness routine—is to listen to your body. It will tell you what it wants and does not want. Be aware, though, that when your body is full of toxins, it is going to tell you that it wants more of the offending foods. That's the definition of a craving! Your body becomes dependent on toxic foods. As you cleanse, you'll find that your body will start to desire healthier foods, and it will be easier to trust the signals that it gives you.

And for you sugarholics and carbaholics, there is good news. Once you start to eradicate fungus and balance out blood sugar levels, your cravings for sugar and carbs will subside, making it that much easier to adhere to the program.

FOODS TO EAT

As you look at the lists that follow, you will see other foods that may cause inflammation or an allergy response. While you don't necessarily need to eliminate these foods for 90 days, you do need to eliminate them for a significant period to allow your body to return to homeostasis. In the lists below, I have designated the appropriate amount of time to refrain from each of the offending foods.

Animal protein (antibiotic- and hormone-free as much as possible; eat 2–4 ounces daily or no less than three times a week)

- Beef, bison, lamb, venison (grass-fed; no more than a 3- to 4-ounce serving once a week; prepare rare to medium-rare and eat with greens and not with starchy vegetables, beans, or grains)
- Chicken, duck, turkey
- Chicken and turkey hot dogs and sausages (nitrate-, hormone-, and gluten-free)
- Eggs (organic or pasture-raised, if possible)
- Fish (limit shellfish to once or twice a month)
- Turkey bacon (nitrate-, hormone-, and gluten-free)

Grains (whole and unrefined only)

- Amaranth
- Breads (gluten-, yeast-, sugar-, and dairy-free)
- Brown rice (short- and long-grain, brown basmati; limit to 2–3 times a week)
- Brown rice cakes and crackers (limit to 2–3 times a week)
- Buckwheat
- Millet
- Oats (gluten-free, only after two months on the program)*
- Pasta (brown-rice, buckwheat, quinoa pasta only; limit to once a week)
- Quinoa
- Sorghum (can make like popcorn)
- Tapioca
- Teff
- Wild rice
- Yucca

*Oats do not contain gluten; however, they are sometimes cross-contaminated with other gluten grains. Therefore, when eating oats, purchase a brand that ensures that it is gluten-free, such as Bob's Red Mill.

Vegetables

All vegetables may be eaten, except corn, mushrooms, peas, and potatoes. Eating fresh mushrooms can create an allergy response (histamine reaction) and slow down positive results in the first 90 days of your program.

Limit sweet potatoes, yams, and winter squash to up to 3 servings a week total. Limit or avoid nightshade-family vegetables (eggplant, tomatoes, potatoes, and peppers) for the first 90 days, because they can cause inflammation. If you eat them and your symptoms increase, avoid completely for the first three months and then reintroduce in small amounts if you wish.

Beans and Legumes

You may eat small quantities once or twice a week only or avoid this group entirely for the first two months of the program because of their potential to cause inflammation and their high starch levels, which raise blood sugar. If you avoid them and then reintroduce, eat only small amounts once or twice weekly. In either case, do not eat any soy, fermented soy products, or peas. Bragg Liquid Aminos is the only soy product allowed and may be used from the beginning of your program.

Nuts and Seeds (raw; unroasted if commercial; may dry-roast your own)

- Almonds
- Brazil nuts
- Chestnuts
- Chia seeds
- Flaxseed
- Hazelnuts
- Hempseed
- Macadamia nuts
- Nut butters (almond and macadamia only; may be raw or dry-roasted)
- Pecans
- Pili nuts
- Pine nuts
- Pumpkin seeds and pumpkin-seed butter
- Sesame seeds (also raw tahini butter)
- Sunflower seeds and sunflower-seed butter
- Walnuts

Note: Limit quantities of nuts and seeds to a small handful at a time, and chew thoroughly.

Oils (cold-pressed only)

Almond oil (can be used for cooking)

Avocado oil (can be used for cooking)

Coconut oil (can be used for cooking)

Flaxseed oil (not for cooking)

Grapeseed oil (can be used for cooking)

Hempseed oil (not for cooking)

Olive oil (can be used for cooking)

Pistachio oil (not for cooking; after 90 days)

Red palm fruit oil (can be used for cooking, low heat only)

Sesame oil (can be used for cooking)

Sunflower oil (can be used for cooking)

Walnut oil (not for cooking)

Dairy (antibiotic- and hormone-free only)

Butter (small amounts, unsalted, preferably pasture-raised organic from grass-fed cows)

Clarified butter (ghee, organic pasture-raised)

Goat cheese (raw; small amounts after 90 days)*

Sheep cheese (raw; small amounts after 90 days)*

*Pregnant and nursing women should not eat raw dairy products.

Fruits (organic; no dried fruit or fruit juices)†

Apples (only green apples for first 90 days)

Avocado‡

Blackberries (discard if you see any visible mold)

Blueberries (discard if you see any visible mold)

Coconut flesh and/or unsweetened milk (no coconut juice or coconut water)

Cranberries (fresh, unsweetened)

Grapefruit

Lemons, limes‡

Olives (without vinegar or preservatives only)

Raspberries (discard if you see any visible mold)

Strawberries (discard if you see any visible mold)

†Limit fruit intake to one piece per day, about the size of a medium apple in volume, or a handful of berries.

‡Avocado serving and lemon or lime juice may be in addition to your one fruit per day.

Condiments

Apple cider vinegar (raw, unfiltered only—refrigerate)

Bragg Liquid Aminos (unfermented soy sauce; only acceptable soy product)

Coconut Aminos (soy-free seasoning sauce)

Dill relish (Bubbies brand, made without vinegar only; after 90 days)

Dry mustard (or small amounts of mustard made with apple cider vinegar)

Fresh herbs (basil, parsley, etc.)

Healthy Mayonnaise (see recipe, page 179)

Himalayan salt

Kelp flakes (Bragg Organic Sea Kelp Delight Seasoning)

Pepper

Sea salt

Spices (without sugar, MSG, or additives); favor ginger and turmeric, which are anti-inflammatory)

Beverages

Bragg apple cider vinegar drinks (Ginger Spice, Limeade, and Sweet Stevia only)

Herbal teas (red clover, peppermint, chamomile, etc.)

Organic white tea (caffeinated)

Suja Lemon Love (lemon juice drink)

Unsweetened almond, Brazil nut, coconut, and hemp milk

Unsweetened mineral water

Water (filtered, purified, or distilled only)

Sweeteners

Chicory root (Just Like Sugar)

Lo han kuo (monk fruit extract, also known as luo han guo)

Stevia (Kal liquid)

Xylitol, in small amounts (Ultimate Sweetener or Xyla brands)

Miscellaneous

Cacao powder (raw, unsweetened; small amounts after 2 months)

Carob (unsweetened; small amounts after 2 months because it is an inflammatory legume)

Cocoa powder (unsweetened; small amounts after 2 months)

Coconut butter (organic)

Dill pickles (made without vinegar only, such as Bubbies brand; after 90 days)

Gums/mints (sweetened with lo han, stevia, or xylitol)

Salsa (without sugar or vinegar, except apple cider vinegar)

Sauerkraut (made without vinegar only, such as Bubbies brand; after 90 days)

FOODS TO AVOID

Avoid the foods on this list while you are on the anti-candida diet. After 90 days (unless a different time period is specified), you may include the foods marked with an asterisk (*). Add one food at a time every third day and see if your body reacts—if you experience rapid heartbeat, itching, bloating and gas, constipation, fatigue, or worsening of your symptoms. If this happens, keep these foods out of your diet for another three months and then try again if you wish.

Animal Protein

Bacon

Hot dogs

Pork

Processed and packaged meats

Sausage

Tuna (all: toro, albacore, ahi, etc., including canned)

Grains

Barley

Breads (except those that are gluten-, dairy-, yeast-, and sugar-free and do not contain the grains listed here)

Cereals (except gluten-, dairy-, and sugar-free)

Corn (tortillas, polenta, popcorn, chips, etc.)

Crackers (except gluten-, dairy-, yeast-, and sugar-free; do not eat any with corn, potato, and/or white flour)

Farro

Kamut

Oats* (use gluten-free after 2 months)

Pasta (except those made from brown rice, buckwheat, and quinoa)

Pastries

Rye

Spelt

Triticale

Wheat (refined)

White flours
White rice
Whole wheat

Vegetables

Corn
Mushrooms
Peas*
Potatoes

Beans and Legumes

You may eat small amounts once or twice a week or avoid these entirely for the first 2 months of the program because of their potential to cause inflammation and their high starch levels, which raise blood sugar. If you avoid them and then reintroduce, eat small amounts once or twice a week only, but continue to stay off soy (tofu, soybeans, tamari, and ponzu sauce) and fermented soy products (miso, tempeh, etc.).

Nuts and Seeds

Cashews*
Peanuts, peanut butter
Pistachios*

Oils

Canola oil
Corn oil
Cottonseed oil
Peanut oil
Pistachio oil*
Processed oils and partially hydrogenated or hydrogenated oils
Soy oil

Dairy

Buttermilk
Cheeses (al including cottage and cream cheese)
Cow's milk
Goat's milk and cheese (raw okay after 90 days, small amounts)*

Ice cream
Margarine
Sheep cheese (raw okay after 90 days, small amounts)*
Sour cream
Yogurt

Note: Pregnant and nursing women should not eat raw dairy products.

Fruits

Apricots*
Bananas*
Cherries*
Cranberries (sweetened)
Dried fruits (all, including apricots, dates, figs, raisins, cranberries, prunes, etc.)
Grapes*
Guavas*
Juices (all, sweetened or unsweetened)
Kiwis*
Mangoes*
Melons*
Nectarines*
Oranges*
Papayas*
Peaches*
Pears*
Persimmons*
Pineapples*
Plums*
Pomegranates*
Tangerines*

Beverages

Alcohol
Caffeinated teas (except white tea)
Coffee (caffeinated and decaffeinated)
Energy drinks (such as Red Bull, vitamin waters)
Fruit juices
Kefir
Kombucha
Rice and soy milks
Sodas (diet and regular)

Condiments

Gravy
Healthy Mayonnaise (see recipe, page 179)
Jams and jellies
Ketchup
Mustard (unless made with apple cider vinegar; small amounts)
Pickles
Relish

Salad dressing (unless sugar-free and made with apple cider vinegar)

Sauces with vinegars and sugar

Soy sauce, ponzu, and tamari sauce

Spices that contain yeast, sugar, or additives

Vinegars (all, except raw, unfiltered apple cider vinegar and unsweetened rice vinegar—keep refrigerated)

Worcestershire sauce

Sweeteners

Agave nectar (Nectevia)

Artificial sweeteners, such as aspartame (Nutrasweet), acesulfame potassium, saccharin, and sucralose (Splenda)

Barley malt

Brown rice syrup

Brown sugar

Coconut sugar/nectar

Corn syrup

Dextrose

Erythritol (Nectresse, Swerve, Truvia)

Fructose, products sweetened with fruit juice

Honey (raw or processed; raw honey may be used medicinally)

Maltitol

Maltodextrin

Mannitol

Maple syrup

Molasses

Raw or evaporated cane juice crystals

Sorbitol

White sugar

Yacon syrup

Miscellaneous

Cacao/chocolate (unless sweetened with stevia or xylitol; small amounts after 2 months)*

Candy

Carob (unsweetened, small amounts after 2 months because it is an inflammatory legume)*

Cookies

Doughnuts

Fast food and fried foods

Fermented foods (kimchi, kombucha, sauerkraut, tempeh, yogurt, nutritional yeast, cultured vegetables, etc.)

Fruit strips

Gelatin

Gum (unless sweetened with stevia or xylitol)

Jerky (beef, turkey)

Lozenges/mints (unless sweetened with lo han, stevia, or xylitol)

Muffins

Pastries
Pizza
Processed food (TV dinners, etc.)
Smoked, dried, pickled, and cured foods

SAMPLE MENUS

The two weeks' worth of sample menus that follow will give you an idea of the diverse menus you can create while on the anti-candida diet. You will find recipes for some of the dishes in the Recipes chapter, which also includes recipes not listed here. Be aware that some of these meals contain foods and ingredients that you may only eat after being on the diet for two or three months, so familiarize yourself with the "Foods to Eat" and "Foods to Avoid" lists.

Week One

Day One

Upon arising	1 cup of red clover tea
Breakfast	Poached egg with side of sautéed vegetables (onions and kale), topped with slices of avocado
Snack	Apple (green) with a small handful of raw almonds
Lunch	Millet Tabouli (page 169)
Snack	Vegetable Alkalizer Juice (page 196) (8 ounces)
Dinner	Baked Salmon over Leafy Greens (page 148)

Day Two

Upon arising	1 cup of red clover tea
Breakfast	Mixed Veggie Quiche (page 132)
Snack	Blueberries topped with coconut butter
Lunch	Arugula, Beet, and Walnut Salad (page 171)
Snack	Jicama slices dipped in Tahini Dressing (page 178)

Dinner	Tuscan Roast Chicken (page 153), Artichoke with Dipping Sauce (page 161), sautéed yellow squash in olive oil and herbs

Day Three

Upon arising	1 cup of red clover tea
Breakfast	Granola (page 138) with berries, unsweetened almond, coconut, or hemp milk
Snack	Cut-up raw vegetables (broccoli, carrots, jicama, asparagus) with Ranch Dressing (page 177)
Lunch	African-Style Turkey (page 158), spinach, red onion, and sprout salad with Italian Vinaigrette Dressing* (page 176)
Snack	Handful of Spicy Almonds, Walnuts, or Pecans (page 191), 1 cup of red clover tea
Dinner	Kelp noodles with garlic, pine nuts, basil, and sautéed vegetables

Day Four

Upon arising	1 cup of red clover tea
Breakfast	Creamy Blueberry-Vanilla Buckwheat Porridge (page 135)
Snack	Vegetable Alkalizer Juice (page 196) (8 ounces)
Lunch	Chicken Stir-Fry (page 149)
Snack	Olive Tapenade (page 181) with flax or almond crackers, 1 cup of red clover tea
Dinner	Thai Spiced Lentil Soup (page 147)

Day Five

Upon arising	1 cup of red clover tea
Breakfast	Egg sandwich (sunny-side-up egg on lettuce or coconut wrap with Healthy Mayonnaise (page 179), sprouts, avocado, and sesame seeds)
Snack	Celery sticks with sunflower-seed butter, 1 cup of red clover tea
Lunch	Chopped Taco Salad (page 173)
Snack	Vegetable Alkalizer Juice (page 196) (8 ounces)

Dinner	Cod with Macadamia Cream Sauce (page 185), Roasted Brussels Sprouts (page 163)

Day Six

Upon arising	2 cups of red clover tea
Breakfast	Blueberry Pancakes (page 136)
Snack	Lemon-Poppyseed Shake (page 197)
Lunch	Quinoa Medley (page 167), Cucumber Salad (page 174)
Snack	Kale Chips (page 192), 1 cup of red clover tea
Dinner	Lamb Burger (page 141) (with mustard, avocado, and sautéed onion) wrapped in lettuce leaf, side of broccoli florets and cucumber slices, with Tahini Dressing (page 178)

Day Seven

Upon arising	2 cups of red clover tea
Breakfast	Vegetable scramble with diced squash, cauliflower, mustard greens, chives, and cooked quinoa
Snack	Guacamole (page 183) with cut-up vegetables
Lunch	Butter Lettuce, Hard-Boiled Egg, and Nutty "Parmesan" (page 171)
Snack	Kale-Ginger Cleanser (page 196)
Dinner	Buckwheat Pizza (page 155), mixed green salad with Italian Vinaigrette Dressing (page 176)
Dessert	Carrot Muffin (page 186), chamomile tea

Week Two

Day One

Upon arising	2 cups of red clover tea
Breakfast	Protein Smoothie (page 198)
Snack	Half a grapefruit

Lunch	Baked trout with Garlic and Cilantro Marinade (page 181), grilled asparagus with toasted sesame seeds, Citrus Soda (page 195)
Snack	Half an avocado with a sprinkle of sea salt, 1 cup of red clover tea
Dinner	Nutty Seed Burger (page 140), Asian Coleslaw (page 175)

Day Two

Upon arising	2 cups of red clover tea
Breakfast	Paleo Pancakes (page 137)
Snack	Vegetable Alkalizer Juice (page 196) (8 ounces)
Lunch	Homemade Chicken Soup (page 146)
Snack	Celery and carrot sticks with Ranch Dressing (page 177), 2 cups of red clover tea
Dinner	Fish Curry (page 149) over Nutty Brown Rice (page 168), Marinated Kale Salad (page 172)

Day Three

Upon arising	2 cups of red clover tea
Breakfast	Arugula salad topped with grilled onions, turkey bacon, and poached egg, drizzled with olive oil, sea salt, and pepper
Snack	Cucumber slices and sprouts with raw apple, cider vinegar, sea salt, and pepper
Lunch	Indian Risotto (page 153)
Snack	Pumpkin seeds (a small handful), 2 cups of red clover tea
Dinner	Herbed Meat Loaf (page 142), Mashed Faux-tatoes (page 159), Spinach Salad (page 175)

Day Four

Upon arising	2 cups of red clover tea
Breakfast	Granola (page 138) with unsweetened coconut, hemp, or almond milk
Snack	Flax crackers with pumpkin-seed butter

Lunch	Spaghetti Squash with Parsley Pesto Sauce (page 143)
Snack	Green apple with a small handful of walnuts, 2 cups of red clover tea
Dinner	Roast Duckling (page 154), Cabbage and Leeks (page 166), Mashed Sweet Potato (page 160)

Day Five

Upon arising	2 cups of red clover tea
Breakfast	Egg Muffins (page 133)
Snack	Garlic-Rosemary Paleo Bread (page 170) with ghee
Lunch	Avocado Salad (page 174)
Snack	Coconut Cream Parfait (page 139), 2 cups of red clover tea
Dinner	Halibut with Olive Tapenade (page 181), Stir-Fried Asparagus (page 161)

Day Six

Upon arising	2 cups of red clover tea
Breakfast	Mixed Berry Waffles (page 139)
Snack	Raw vegetable slices with Herbed "Sour Cream" (page 180)
Lunch	BLT salad (chopped romaine lettuce, diced avocado, sliced tomatoes, cut-up cooked turkey bacon, diced jicama) and Ranch Dressing (page 177)
Snack	Blueberry–Pumpkin Seed Shake (page 197), 2 cups of red clover tea
Dinner	Vegan or Bison Lasagna (page 151), mixed green salad with Cumin Vinaigrette (page 176)

Day Seven

Upon arising	2 cups of red clover tea
Breakfast	Ground chicken with vegetables (diced cauliflower, peppers, garlic, spinach)

Snack	Vegetable Alkalizer Juice (page 196) (8 ounces)
Lunch	Buckwheat Pizza (page 155)
Snack	Southern Greens Mix (page 166), 2 cups of red clover tea
Dinner	Egg Salad (page 145), watercress, fennel, avocado, and sliced green apple salad with Cumin Vinaigrette (page 176)
Dessert	Baked Apple Crumble (page 187)

CONSUMING BEVERAGES

You may have noticed that in the sample food plans, drinks are typically consumed first thing in the morning or as a snack. I don't recommend consuming beverages with meals. When you drink any beverage, even water, you waterlog your digestive enzymes (HCl and pepsin) that break down proteins. Extra liquid inhibits enzyme function and disrupts the digestive process.

Optimal digestion helps promote gut health. When your food isn't properly broken down by digestive enzymes, it will begin fermenting in the gut, providing a food source for candida, bacteria, and parasites. I'm not suggesting that you can't sip a little bit of water with a meal—I don't want you to choke on dry food. But too many people drink sixteen to thirty-two ounces with each meal (especially if drinking soda), and that's way too much.

Meal Ideas

The meal ideas below will show you just some of the possibilities for creating tasty meals while on the anti-candida diet. It's important to have a varied selection of foods so you don't get bored! Limit animal protein to no more than four to eight ounces daily. You will find recipes for some of the dishes in chapter 7, "Delicious Recipes to Beat Candida."

Breakfast Ideas

- Eggs or egg whites prepared in a variety of ways with a side of steamed spinach, squash, cauliflower, or kale (soft-boiled, poached, hard-boiled, and sunny-side-up eggs are best; eat scrambled eggs or omelets infrequently because of oxidized cholesterol from the yolks, or use egg whites only)
- Soft-boiled eggs with avocado
- Omelet with vegetables (asparagus, spinach, and onion)
- Eggs with arugula or spinach: Layer pan with olive oil and a large handful of washed spinach or arugula. Crack eggs on top of greens and cover with a lid; steam until yolks are set as desired.
- Hard-boiled egg with mustard or Basiltops dairy-free pesto
- Egg scramble: Prepare with 2 egg whites, 2–3 spoonfuls of cooked quinoa or wild rice, No-Cheese Pesto (page 180), and a handful of washed kale or spinach (sautéed until tender).
- Brown rice tortillas, heated with ghee, nut butter, coconut butter, or tahini
- Egg sandwich/burrito: poached or sunny-side-up egg, Healthy Mayonnaise (page 179), sliced red onion, and spinach leaves on a heated brown rice tortilla or lettuce leaf
- Hot cereal (amaranth, brown rice, buckwheat, or quinoa) with nuts, flax or chia seeds, berries, a splash of almond, coconut, or hemp milk, and a sprinkle of cinnamon, sweetened with stevia, lo han, or xylitol if desired
- Turkey bacon or chicken sausage (antibiotic-, hormone- and gluten-free; if casing is pork, peel off after cooking) with sautéed vegetables
- Protein smoothie made with egg white or 1 scoop hemp, pumpkin seed, or brown rice protein powder (no sugar), unsweetened almond, coconut, or hemp milk, one piece of fruit from "Foods to Eat" list; handful of spinach or kale, 1 tsp raw almond butter or coconut oil (melted) or raw nuts/seeds from "Foods to Eat" list; and a couple of drops of Kal Pure Stevia liquid (optional).

- Ground turkey or chicken sautéed with diced sweet potatoes and onions
- Cold cereal: Granola (page 138), Lydia's Sprouted Cinnamon Cereal, Go Raw Simple Granola, or Nature's Path Qi'a Superfood—Chia, Buckwheat & Hemp Cereal with almond milk, pecans, berries, and cinnamon, sweetened with stevia, lo han, or xylitol if desired
- Vegetable Alkalizer Juice (page 196), made with organic veggies
- Gluten-free waffles or pancakes (such as Paleo Pancakes, page 137), garnished with sliced almonds and cinnamon
- Amazing Meal Vanilla Chai Infusion (protein drink), mixed with 8 ounces of cold unsweetened almond milk
- Vegetable scramble (arugula, squash, onions, broccoli, and fresh herbs sautéed in olive oil) served over a bed of cooked millet or quinoa

Lunch and Dinner Ideas

- Salad (greens: spinach, arugula, baby greens, and/or watercress; red onion; sprouts; sliced or grated carrots, jicama, radishes, and/or green apple; nuts, etc.) with Italian Vinaigrette Dressing (page 176)
- Black kale salad massaged with fresh lemon juice: Put in the refrigerator for a couple of hours to soften the kale and then add pine nuts, sea salt, and pepper
- BLT salad: chopped romaine lettuce, diced avocado, cut-up cooked turkey bacon, diced jicama, and Ranch Dressing (page 177)
- Cruciferous salad: cut-up spinach, watercress, parsley, avocado, red cabbage, green onions, cauliflower, and/or cucumber, topped with sesame seeds and Italian Vinaigrette Dressing (page 176)
- Raw vegetable salad: shredded beets, zucchini, jicama, and chopped cucumber, topped with alfalfa sprouts and dressing
- Chef's salad: baby greens, tomatoes, and cucumber, with diced cooked turkey, cut-up hard-boiled egg, and dressing
- Greek salad: romaine lettuce, cut-up cooked chicken breast, olives, and lemon-dill dressing

- Brown rice and steamed or sautéed vegetables, drizzled with olive oil, seasoned with sea salt, herbs or spices
- Buckwheat (no wheat) soba or kelp noodles in a stir-fry or with sautéed vegetables or chicken (use cold-pressed sesame oil and Bragg Liquid Aminos)
- Turkey burger with baked Sweet Potato Fries (page 169)
- Steamed vegetables topped with Macadamia Cream Sauce (page 185)
- Broiled, poached, or sautéed fish (salmon, cod, halibut, sole, trout, etc.) with a side of sautéed greens
- Chicken salad on half an avocado
- Stews prepared in a Crock-Pot
- Baked vegetable medley: purple cabbage, kale, onion, red peppers, and Brussels sprouts (toss vegetables in olive oil and herbs before baking), served over cooked millet
- Soups, nondairy and sugar-free (vegetable, chicken vegetable, turkey, leek-broccoli puree, cauliflower-celery, carrot-celery-ginger, parsnip-butternut squash, etc.)
- Brown rice or quinoa pasta with fresh tomatoes, pine nuts, olive oil, garlic, and other vegetables if desired
- BLT wrap (cut-up cooked turkey bacon, lettuce, tomato, and avocado, with a small amount of Healthy Mayonnaise, page 179) in a brown rice tortilla or lettuce leaf
- Turkey chili with a side of mixed green salad (small amounts because of the beans)
- Stuffed zucchini or peppers (ground chicken or turkey, chopped onion, and seasonings) topped with marinara sauce
- Chicken or turkey tacos in brown rice tortillas or lettuce leaf, with guacamole, salsa, and shredded lettuce
- Chicken (broiled, roasted, baked, poached) with sautéed kale, cauliflower, and Brussels sprouts
- Lamb Burger (page 141) or beef steak with sautéed onions, with a side of sautéed asparagus

- Chicken or turkey sausage cut up and dipped in mustard, with a side salad
- Vegetable stir-fry with or without chicken or fish (use cold-pressed sesame oil and Coconut Aminos)
- Roast chicken prepared with fresh herbs (thyme, rosemary), with a side of roasted vegetables (purple cabbage, carrots, peppers, onions, kale—toss veggies in olive oil and seasoning before roasting)
- Turkey dogs (no nitrates, sugar, or dairy) with oven-baked turnip or parsnip fries (toss in grapeseed oil before baking)
- Turkey or chicken sandwich on gluten-, yeast-, dairy-, and sugar-free bread or lettuce wrap, with avocado, spinach, and mustard
- Egg salad sandwich on Garlic-Rosemary Paleo Bread (page 170) or lettuce wrap (use Healthy Mayonnaise, page 179)
- Lettuce wraps filled with diced chicken salad, wild rice, and slivered almonds
- Seaweed wraps filled with wild rice, chopped vegetable medley, and freshly grated ginger (use organic nori sheets)

Side Dish Ideas

- Shredded slaw salad (raw purple and green cabbage and carrots with raw apple cider vinegar and seasonings)
- Collard greens or black kale sautéed in olive oil, with a splash of raw apple cider vinegar
- Sliced cucumbers with raw apple cider vinegar and sea salt
- Wild rice pilaf made with organic chicken broth (no sugar)
- Mashed sweet potatoes or cauliflower made with almond milk and olive oil
- Artichoke with Dipping Sauce (page 161), or melted butter, or Healthy Mayonnaise (page 179)
- Swiss chard, chopped and sautéed in olive oil, with pine nuts, fresh herbs, and sea salt
- Sautéed onions, peppers, and squashes

- Cold brown rice salad with raw apple cider vinegar, vegetables, and seasonings
- Parsnips with butter (puree in blender)
- Asparagus sautéed in toasted sesame oil and sprinkled with sesame seeds
- Baked butternut squash with a small amount of butter and stevia
- Quinoa with seasonings and spices or Basiltops dairy-free pesto or No-Cheese Pesto (page 180)
- Baked Brussels sprouts and cauliflower with garlic, sea salt, and olive oil
- Millet with herbs and olive oil or Parsley Pesto Sauce (page 179)
- Steamed broccoli and cauliflower with melted ghee or butter
- Amaranth with butter and seasonings
- Onions sautéed in olive oil, fresh thyme, sea salt, and pepper
- Oven-baked turnip fries (toss in grapeseed oil before baking)
- Brown basmati rice sautéed in olive oil with cumin, topped with pine nuts or sliced almonds
- Fresh sprouts (broccoli, radish, sunflower) with fresh lemon juice or raw apple cider vinegar
- Radish and fennel salad with fresh dill and raw apple cider vinegar
- Oven-roasted vegetables (squash, onions, carrots, red cabbage) seasoned with thyme and rosemary (toss in olive oil before roasting)

Snacks and Desserts

- Gluten-Free Crepes (page 188) with almond or coconut butter or sesame seed tahini, a drop of stevia, and a sprinkle of cinnamon
- Hard-boiled egg with mustard
- Kale Chips (page 192)
- Almond crackers or flax crackers with nut/seed butter (almond, macadamia nut, sunflower seed, or pumpkin seed) or coconut butter

- Steve's Original Paleo Stix (grass-fed beef sticks from Steve's PaleoGoods)
- Cut-up vegetables (carrot sticks, broccoli, jicama, celery) dipped in Tahini Dressing (page 178), Ranch Dressing (page 177), or Guacamole (page 183)
- Garlic spread (Majestic Garlic) on Jilz Gluten Free Crackerz or on crusts (Mauk Family Farms' Raw Wheat Free or Raw Mineral Rich Crusts)
- Celery with almond butter, macadamia nut butter, sunflower-seed butter, or pumpkin-seed butter
- Fruit from the "Foods to Eat" list, one piece (or a handful of berries)
- Kabocha Squash Slices (page 164)
- Baked apple with cinnamon and nuts
- Cookies and treats made without gluten, dairy, or sugar (such as Nutty Nibbles by Nut Just a Cookie, sugar-free variety). Or make your own, using gluten-free flours; coconut flour; almond meal; butter, ghee, or coconut oil; nut butters; and sweeteners such as stevia, lo han, chicory root, or xylitol.
- Smoothie made with egg-white or pumpkin-seed protein powder, almond milk, blueberries, and nut butter (or melted coconut oil or coconut butter); see Blueberry–Pumpkin Seed Shake (page 197)
- Cacao bars (Rox Chox, made with xylitol; after two months)

Sauces and Seasonings

- Salsa (page 183) (no sugar or vinegar, except raw apple cider vinegar)
- Guacamole (page 183) (avocados, tomatoes, onion, and spices)
- Sesame-ginger-garlic sauce, made with cold-pressed sesame oil, ginger, and garlic
- Lemon-garlic sauce, made with olive oil, garlic, and lemon juice (use over gluten-free pasta)

- Fresh-squeezed lemon or lime juice
- Bragg Liquid Aminos (unfermented soy sauce; salty flavor is good for stir-fries)
- Italian Vinaigrette Dressing (page 176)
- Unsweetened orange or pineapple juice as a marinade for fish or chicken (these fruits are acceptable only for marinade)
- Healthy Mayonnaise (page 179)
- Bragg Organic Sea Kelp Delight Seasoning
- Seaweed flakes
- Curry (coconut milk, turmeric, cumin, ginger, and garlic paste)
- Raw Coconut Aminos (use like soy sauce; coconutsecret.com)
- Macadamia Cream Sauce (page 185)
- Spices—cayenne, turmeric, ginger, cumin, epazote, coriander, curry, cinnamon, bay leaves, basil, and others

Eating Out

After looking through the food lists, you might worry that you won't be able to eat out or enjoy social gatherings on this plan. But I assure you, this is not the case—there is always an easy workaround. The key is to just do the best you can. If you find yourself at a restaurant and the only protein served is barbecued chicken, just scrape off the sauce and eat the chicken. If you're at a party and all they're serving is pizza and salad with balsamic vinegar, choose the salad with the balsamic vinegar. If only sandwiches are served, throw away both slices of the bread and eat what's inside.

It helps to understand that these dietary changes are not about deprivation—they are about eating foods that will not feed yeast to help restore your health. If you slip up and eat something that's not on the plan, don't let guilt take over. Negative emotions are not only bad for your mental and physical health, but on a practical level, they can also prevent you from making positive choices that support your long-term goals.

As it was the holidays when I was compiling new information for this book, I checked in with several clients to see how they were handling the traditional family gatherings. Many of them used the strategy of bringing a dish of their own to a party, potluck-style, so they knew there would be at least one thing there they could eat. Others ate beforehand, so they could nibble on something small at the party that fit the anti-candida protocol. And some had their families and friends make a dish or two that they *could* eat.

That said, there will be occasions in which you want to indulge a little, and that's fine. Some of the most common "cheats" are alcohol, sweet treats, carb-y snacks and bread, and dairy foods. Believe it or not, not all these offenders are equally damaging. In fact, alcoholic beverages, particularly wine, beer, and champagne, do the most damage. Alcohol is a double threat: it's liquid sugar to the body, plus it's fermented, or yeasty if you are drinking wine, beer, sake, or champagne. If you indulge in alcohol, I advise drinking vodka with club soda and fresh lemon/lime, since it is distilled and has no sugar. The second most damaging cheat is refined sugar—that is, brownies, cookies, pastries, ice cream, and so on. Third is gluten, which is commonly found in white flour products like crackers, pasta, breads, and pizza. And the fourth setback food is dairy. With this in mind, you can choose your indulgences wisely. It's actually better to cheat with a nice piece of fresh cheese than it is to drink a glass of wine, dip into that pasta salad, or have a brownie!

When you have indulged in alcohol or sugar, or consumed another food that's not on the plan, I recommend drinking three or four cups of red clover tea or one or two cups of white tea to help clear the toxins from your bloodstream. But don't abuse this workaround—it isn't the same as eating cleanly. If you indulge frequently, you won't experience the results you're looking for.

Most of All, Don't Give Up

Beating candida requires both patience and discipline. If you stick to the diet and supplement program between 80 and 100 percent of the time, you will assure your success. Slipping below 80 percent doesn't mean you won't feel better, but it does mean your progress will be slower.

Make it easier on yourself by shopping at health food stores and online sites such as amazon.com, vitacost.com, iherb.com, thrive market.com, and websites for the healthy products listed in my book. Not only will you find many wonderful choices but you will also be eating more health-giving, nutritious foods. Wherever you shop, be sure to carefully read labels, as even "health foods" sometimes contain sugar and ingredients you need to avoid while on the anti-candida diet.

Strict monitoring of your diet is essential. However, if you've had a bad day and eaten something that's not on your diet, don't beat yourself up; just get back into your regimen and keep going. Persevere, and the results will come. You'll notice improvements in your health in as little as two to four weeks, and experience even greater changes after two to three months.

It's best to approach getting rid of candida overgrowth as a lifestyle change rather than as a temporary fix. Once you feel better, you'll find that you are more sensitive to how food affects your body and mind because you are conscious of it, and you won't even want to go back to making poor food choices. As my client Janet said, "Now that I've dumped the sugar—all of it, fruit, dairy, grain, and legumes—I've seen such improvement, and I feel too good to eat the old food anymore."

The Five-Week Slow-Start Modified Plan

Those who would prefer to ease into the candida elimination program can follow a slower schedule, gradually eliminating the offending foods week by week over a period of five weeks. Once you have successfully eliminated all the foods on the following lists, you are ready to begin your first month of the 90-day program to eliminate candida and detoxify your body, as outlined in chapters 6 and 7.

Note that some of the foods on these lists may be reintroduced after you've been on the program for two or three months. Check the "Foods to Avoid" list on page 108 for more details.

Week One

Eliminate dairy products (less dairy leads to less mucus and inflammation)

Eliminate cigarettes and recreational drugs

Week Two

Eliminate refined carbohydrates and gluten (fewer refined carbohydrates means less pain and inflammation, as well as improved weight loss)

Week Three

Eliminate sugar (less sugar means less pain and inflammation and improved weight loss). Sugar includes refined sugar, artificial sweeteners, and natural sugars such as cane sugar, agave nectar, coconut nectar/sugar, molasses, maple syrup, and honey.

Week Four

Eliminate alcohol, caffeine, and decaffeinated black tea and coffee.

Also eliminate the following miscellaneous foods:

- Nuts: Cashews, pistachios, peanuts
- Condiments: All ketchup, relish, pickles, etc.
- Vegetables: Mushrooms, potatoes (mushrooms can create an allergy response; potatoes convert rapidly into sugar)
- Beans and legumes (peas and soy)
- All fermented foods (kombucha, kefir, miso, tempeh, soy sauce)
- All processed/fast foods
- All smoked, cured, dried, and pickled foods (bacon, bologna, smoked salmon)

Week Five

Eliminate fruits not on the "Foods to Eat" list (less sugar means less inflammation and increased energy):

- All fruits (except lemons, limes, grapefruit, Granny Smith apples, and coconuts)
- All dried fruits (cranberries, dates, figs, raisins, prunes, etc.)
- All fruit juices (sweetened and unsweetened)

ENCOURAGEMENT FROM MEGHAN

It was hard giving up bananas because I was used to them, but Ann inspired me to try new fruits and vegetables I'd never heard of. Going through the lists makes it seem possible. Now my energy is back up. I'm sleeping better. My weight is totally normalized. I've been getting compliments on how good I look—I'm just more healthy and happy, and not bloated.

7

Delicious Recipes to Beat Candida

Your 90-Day Program

Now that you know which foods to eat and which foods to avoid, let's get cooking.

In this chapter, you'll find a variety of delicious recipes that fit within the parameters of your anti-candida diet. At first you may want to follow the instructions to the letter, but as you get more comfortable with your new diet, you can simply use the recipes here as inspiration for your own creations.

My client Irina observed, "Once I start eating a food that I didn't find particularly appealing before—once I start working it into my own recipes—I'm surprised at how my taste evolves. The biggest example for me is when I discovered that in the morning, hot broth can be as eye-opening and refreshing as coffee."

Remember that the quality of your food matters. Be mindful of your protein sources; whenever possible, select free-range, antibiotic-free, and hormone-free beef, chicken, turkey, and eggs. Buy wild-caught fish instead of farmed, and purchase organic vegetables and fruits. Avoid genetically modified foods. (Unless it's specified on the label, you can generally assume that packaged food products, or the ingredients they're made with, are made from genetically modified foods. Make sure your mustard is made with apple cider vinegar rather than other types, and use purified water for cooking. Whenever a recipe calls for olive oil, use cold-pressed organic extra-virgin olive oil. Finally, please be aware that sweeteners should not be used until you have strictly adhered to the plan for two to three months. Xylitol powder (Ultimate Sweetener, from Ultimate Life, or Xyla), chicory root (Just Like Sugar), or lo han kuo (Lo Han Sweet, from Jarrow Formulas) may be substituted for stevia (Kal Pure Stevia liquid), if you prefer.

NOT A COOK? NOT A PROBLEM!

You don't have to cook to reap the benefits of this program. Many clients are in professions where they eat out and travel the majority of the time or plain just don't like to cook. When eating out, look for simply prepared meals that consist of animal protein and vegetables. These days, it's easier than ever to both find healthy options in restaurants and to ask for simple modifications when ordering your food. When you find yourself at home, one way to make delicious meals without having to "cook" is to whip up a few of the sauces and keep them in the fridge. Add them to vegetables, salads, and whole grains, or drizzle over proteins like chicken or fish.

Breakfast Dishes

Arugula, Red Onion, and Avocado Frittata

6 servings

6–7 eggs
2 tablespoons filtered water
½ teaspoon sea salt, divided
1 tablespoon olive oil or grass-fed butter for sautéing
¼ cup red onion, diced
½ cup packed arugula
½ avocado, diced small
Pinch black pepper

Preheat oven to broil. In a medium mixing bowl, whisk together the eggs, water, and ¼ teaspoon salt and set aside.

Place olive oil or butter in a well-seasoned 12-inch cast-iron skillet over medium heat and sauté the diced red onions and remaining ¼ teaspoon sea salt for a couple of minutes. Add the arugula and avocado and give it a quick stir. Pour the egg mixture into the pan and stir one more time. Cook for about 4–5 minutes, or until the egg mixture starts to set on the bottom.

Using an oven mitt, remove the skillet from the burner and place in the oven to broil for about 4–5 minutes, or until lightly browned and fluffy. Remove from the oven and let cool for a couple of minutes before slicing.

Mixed Veggie Quiche

6 servings

For the Crust

Olive oil spray

1½ cups almond meal

⅓ cup brown rice flour

½ teaspoon sea salt

Pinch black pepper

2 tablespoons water

⅓ cup olive oil

For the Filling

7–8 organic, free-range eggs

2 tablespoons filtered water or nondairy milk

½ teaspoon sea salt, divided

2 tablespoons olive oil

4 garlic cloves, minced

¼ cup red onion, diced small

¼ cup butternut squash, small cubes

¼ cup broccoli, chopped

Pinch black pepper

To make the crust: Preheat oven to 400°F. Place baking sheet on the middle rack. Grease a pie dish generously with olive oil spray and set aside. In a medium bowl place the almond meal, brown rice flour, sea salt, and pepper and sift using a whisk.

In a separate small bowl, mix the water and oil. Pour the wet ingredients over the dry and combine. Pat this batter into the greased pie dish using your hands to spread evenly around the bottom of the dish and also up the sides. The crust should be about ⅛–¼ inch thick. Poke the entire crust with a fork to prevent bubbles when baking.

Place in the oven and bake until the crust is lightly golden, about 12–15 minutes. Remove from the oven and let cool for about 5–10 minutes before pouring the egg mixture on top.

To make the filling: Reduce heat to 350°F and in a large bowl whisk together the eggs with water or nondairy milk and ¼ teaspoon sea salt. Set aside.

Heat the olive oil in a skillet over medium heat and add the minced garlic and onions with ⅛ teaspoon of sea salt. Sauté for a couple minutes, until the onions start to soften. Next add the butternut squash and broccoli and the remaining ⅛ teaspoon of sea salt and sauté for a couple minutes more.

Place the vegetable mixture in the bowl with the eggs, add a pinch of black pepper, and stir to combine. Finally pour everything into your prepared crust and bake again for 30–35 minutes, or until the center is firm to the touch. Remove from oven and let cool for about 10 minutes before cutting.

Egg Muffins

12 muffins

- 6 strips turkey bacon
- 2 tablespoons olive oil
- ½ cup yellow onion, diced small
- ½ cup red bell pepper, diced small
- ½ teaspoon sea salt, divided
- Pinch black pepper
- 8 eggs
- 2 tablespoons nondairy milk
- 1 scallion, green part only, minced
- 2 tablespoons cilantro, minced

Preheat oven to 350° F. Line a baking sheet with parchment paper and line up turkey bacon strips, being careful not to stack them; bake for about 10–15 minutes, or until cooked. Take a 12-muffin tin, line with silicone liners, and spray generously with oil spray.

In the meantime heat a skillet over medium heat and add olive oil, onion, bell pepper, ¼ teaspoon sea salt, and black pepper and sauté for about 2–3 minutes. Transfer this mixture to a bowl. Whisk together your eggs with the nondairy milk and ¼ teaspoon sea salt. Next add your cooked veggies, as well as the scallion and cilantro.

Once the bacon is done and cooled slightly, chop it into bite-size pieces and add it to your egg mixture. Pour this into 12 muffin cups and bake for 20–25 minutes, or until fully cooked.

Eggs Over Easy with Sautéed Kale

1 serving

- 2 tablespoons grass-fed butter, divided
- 2 room-temperature eggs
- ¼ teaspoon sea salt, divided
- Pinch black pepper
- 2 cups kale, chopped
- 1 teaspoon apple cider vinegar
- ½ avocado, sliced

Heat a nonstick skillet over medium heat with 1 tablespoon of butter. Once butter is warm, crack eggs into the skillet. Sprinkle with ⅛ teaspoon sea salt. Once the white is no longer opaque, using a spatula, gently flip your eggs and cook for about 1 minute more. Carefully remove the eggs from the skillet and sprinkle with pepper.

Next, in the same skillet add 1 more tablespoon of butter and over medium heat add kale, apple cider vinegar, and ⅛ teaspoon sea salt and sauté until the kale has wilted slightly. Pour this onto a plate, and top with eggs and sliced avocado.

Raspberry Quinoa Porridge

2 servings

1 cup white quinoa, uncooked and rinsed
3 cups coconut milk, unsweetened
1 teaspoon vanilla
¼ teaspoon sea salt
1 tablespoon xylitol
5 drops liquid stevia
½ cup fresh raspberries
2 tablespoons flaxseed

In a small saucepan with a fitted lid place the quinoa, coconut milk, vanilla, sea salt, xylitol, and stevia and bring to a boil. Reduce the heat to low, cover, and simmer for about 20 minutes. At this point quinoa is cooked. If you would like the porridge creamier, add more coconut milk; otherwise stir in the raspberries and flaxseed and serve.

Creamy Blueberry-Vanilla Buckwheat Porridge

2 servings

1 cup untoasted buckwheat groats, soaked 4–6 hours in filtered water if possible
3 cups unsweetened vanilla coconut milk
⅓ cup blueberries
1 teaspoon vanilla extract
2–3 tablespoons xylitol (depending on your desired sweetness)
1–5 drops liquid stevia
Pinch sea salt

Rinse the buckwheat in a fine-mesh strainer until the water runs clear. Rinse again if soaking and place in a large saucepan with 3 cups coconut milk, blueberries, vanilla, xylitol, stevia, and a pinch of sea salt. Bring to a boil, reduce to low, and cover. Let simmer for about 20–25 minutes, stirring occasionally. Add more coconut milk if necessary.

Blueberry Pancakes

4 servings

For the Blueberry-Coconut "Syrup"
Zest and juice of 1 lemon
¼ cup coconut cream
¼ cup blueberries, fresh
⅛ teaspoon sea salt
6 drops liquid stevia

1 cup brown rice flour
⅓ cup plus 3 tablespoons tapioca flour
2 tablespoons xylitol
1½ teaspoons baking powder
½ teaspoon baking soda
½ teaspoon sea salt
½ teaspoon xanthan gum
2 eggs
1 teaspoon vanilla extract
1¼ cups unsweetened almond milk
3 tablespoons grapeseed oil
½ cup fresh blueberries
Coconut oil spray for skillet

To make the blueberry-coconut "syrup": Place all ingredients in a blender or food processor and combine.

In a medium bowl mix the rice flour, tapioca flour, xylitol, baking powder, baking soda, sea salt, and xanthan gum. In a separate bowl combine the eggs, vanilla, almond milk, and grapeseed oil, and add to the dry ingredients. Stir until all are combined and there are no lumps. Gently stir in the blueberries.

Heat a skillet or griddle over medium-low heat. Spray generously with coconut oil spray and pour about ¼ cup batter at a time onto the skillet. Cook each side for about 1–2 minutes, until golden brown. Top with blueberry-coconut "syrup."

Paleo Pancakes

Makes about 16 pancakes, or 4 servings

- 1 cup almond flour (not meal)
- ¾ cup tapioca starch
- ¼ cup coconut flour
- 2 teaspoons baking powder
- 2 tablespoons xylitol or 10 drops liquid stevia
- 4 eggs
- 2 tablespoons grapeseed oil
- 1 teaspoon vanilla extract
- ½ cup unsweetened applesauce
- 1 cup almond milk
- ½ cup berries of choice, plus more for serving
- 4 tablespoons grass-fed butter, for cooking
- 3 tablespoons raw almond butter, for serving

Mix almond flour, tapioca starch, coconut flour, baking powder, and xylitol (if using) in a large bowl. In a separate bowl combine stevia (if using), eggs, grapeseed oil, vanilla, applesauce, and almond milk. Next pour wet ingredients into dry ingredients and mix until there are no lumps. Gently stir in your berries.

Heat a nonstick skillet or griddle and grease with your butter. Once the skillet or griddle is hot, pour about ¼ cup batter at a time onto the griddle and cook for about 2 minutes. Gently flip your pancake and cook for about 1 minute more. Serve with almond butter and additional berries.

Granola

4–6 servings

- ¾ cup unsweetened shredded coconut
- 1½ cups slivered almonds
- 1½ cups pecans
- 1 cup walnuts
- 2 tablespoons flaxseed
- 2 tablespoons chia seeds
- 3 tablespoons xylitol
- 1 teaspoon cinnamon
- ¼ cup coconut oil
- 1 teaspoon vanilla extract

Preheat your oven to 300°F. Place rack in the center of the oven. Line a large baking sheet with parchment paper and lightly grease. In a large mixing bowl mix together shredded coconut, slivered almonds, pecans, walnuts, flaxseed, chia seeds, xylitol, and cinnamon.

In a small saucepan over low heat, warm coconut oil and vanilla to bring coconut oil back to liquid state. If coconut oil is already in liquid form, you can skip this part and just mix liquids in a bowl. Next, combine wet ingredients with dry and mix until everything is thoroughly coated. Pour granola onto baking sheet evenly and bake for 12 minutes. Remove from heat, give it a quick stir, and bake for about 12 minutes more, or until it is starting to turn golden brown and is fragrant. Let this cool completely. Store in an airtight container in the refrigerator for one week. Enjoy as a snack or serve for breakfast.

Coconut Cream Parfait

3 servings

1 14-ounce can full-fat coconut cream, solid state
¼ teaspoon vanilla extract
3 tablespoons chia seeds
10 drops liquid stevia or 1 tablespoon xylitol
Pinch sea salt
¼ cup fresh blueberries
¼ cup fresh strawberries, sliced
2 tablespoons slivered almonds
2 tablespoons unsweetened shredded coconut

Place coconut cream, vanilla, chia seeds, stevia or xylitol, and sea salt in a food processor and mix until fully combined. Pour this into a container with a fitted lid and let set in the fridge for about 30–60 minutes. To assemble, place a layer of coconut cream, a layer of berries, and then a sprinkle of almonds and shredded coconut; repeat this one more time. Serve immediately.

Mixed Berry Waffles

4–5 servings

¾ cup brown rice flour
¼ cup almond meal
¼ cup plus 2 tablespoons tapioca flour
1 teaspoon baking powder
⅛ teaspoon sea salt
2 tablespoons xylitol or 10–12 drops liquid stevia
¾ cup coconut milk, unsweetened
2 tablespoons grapeseed oil
2 eggs
¾ cup blackberries; reserve a few for garnish
¾ cup raspberries; reserve a few for garnish
Coconut oil spray for waffle iron
Blueberry-Coconut "Syrup" (page 136)

Preheat waffle iron. In a large mixing bowl, whisk together the brown rice flour, almond meal, tapioca flour, baking powder, sea salt, and xylitol (if using) and mix until well combined and free of lumps. If using stevia, you will add it later.

In a separate bowl, whisk together coconut milk, grapeseed oil, eggs, and stevia (if using). Pour the wet ingredients into the dry and mix until completely combined. Gently stir the blackberries and raspberries into the batter.

For each waffle, spray the heated waffle iron surface with coconut oil spray. Pour the batter, about ⅓ cup at a time, into the center of the waffle iron and cook according to your iron's instructions. Gently remove waffles from the iron. Top with extra berries and serve with the blueberry-coconut syrup.

Main Dishes

Nutty Seeded Burgers

8–10 patties, depending on size

- Coconut oil, for spraying
- 1 cup raw sunflower seeds, soaking optional
- 1 cup raw walnuts, soaking optional
- ¼ cup sun-dried tomatoes in oil
- 1 cup grated carrot
- ½ teaspoon sea salt
- 2 tablespoons fresh parsley, minced
- 2 tablespoons green onions, minced
- 1 teaspoon dried Italian herbs
- ½ teaspoon garlic powder
- 3 tablespoons olive oil

For Serving

8 lettuce wraps

1 avocado, sliced

1 beefsteak tomato, sliced

Red onion slices

Preheat oven to 350°F. Line a baking sheet with foil and spray with coconut oil. Rinse the sunflower seeds and walnuts to clean any dust or debris, place them in a food processor with the remaining ingredients, and blend until a smooth batter is formed. You may have to scrape down the sides occasionally. Taste for seasoning.

Form the batter into patties and place on your prepared baking sheet. Bake patties for about 10–15 minutes, or until they look golden brown. Remove from tray and let cool on a cooling rack. Serve each burger on a lettuce wrap and top with avocado, tomato, and red onion.

Lamb Burger

Makes 4 quarter-pound patties or 8 smaller servings

1 pound ground lamb

¼ cup red onion, minced

3 garlic cloves, minced

¼ cup basil, minced

2 tablespoons olive oil

½ teaspoon sea salt

⅛ teaspoon black pepper

Preheat the oven to 375°F. Line a baking sheet with foil and spray with oil. Set aside. In a large bowl mix together all of the ingredients using your hands. Form into 4 large or 8 small patties and place on the prepared baking sheet. Bake for 20 minutes depending on the size of patties, or until the internal temperature has reached 160°F. Serve in a lettuce wrap or with sautéed vegetables.

Herbed Meat Loaf

4 servings

1 pound ground organic turkey, bison, or beef
1 egg, beaten
¼ cup red onion, minced
3 garlic cloves, minced
1 tablespoon olive oil
2 tablespoons ground flaxseed
1 teaspoon thyme, minced
1 teaspoon rosemary, minced
¼ teaspoon black pepper
¾ teaspoon sea salt

For the Topping

2 tablespoons plain tomato sauce
5 drops liquid stevia
1 teaspoon Coconut Aminos
1 teaspoon apple cider vinegar
⅛ teaspoon sea salt
Pinch black pepper

Preheat oven to 350°F and lightly grease an 8½-by-4½-inch loaf pan. In a large mixing bowl combine meat, egg, red onion, garlic, olive oil, flaxseed meal, thyme, rosemary, pepper, and sea salt until fully combined. Mix with hands. Place into prepared loaf pan. Mix all the ingredients in a bowl and spoon topping over the top of the meat loaf. Bake meat loaf for about 1 hour, or until cooked throughout. Remove meat loaf from the oven and let it cool slightly before removing it from the pan. Slice and serve.

Spaghetti Squash with Parsley Pesto Sauce

2 servings

1 medium organic spaghetti squash
2 tablespoons olive oil, divided
½ teaspoon sea salt, divided
Pinch black pepper
Parsley Pesto Sauce (page 179)
½ cup red onion, sliced into half moons
3 garlic cloves, minced
2 cups loosely packed fresh spinach

Preheat oven to 375°F. Line a baking sheet with parchment paper. Rinse spaghetti squash and cut in half. Scoop out seeds and season with 1 tablespoon olive oil, ¼ teaspoon sea salt, and black pepper. Place on parchment paper, cut side down, and bake for about 40 minutes, or until flesh is tender and yields gently to pressure. While squash is cooking, make Parsley Pesto Sauce.

Next heat a medium skillet over medium-low heat with remaining tablespoon olive oil. Add red onion and garlic and ¼ teaspoon sea salt and sauté for 5 minutes, or until red onion starts to soften. Add spinach, turn off heat, and cover with fitted lid to wilt the spinach. Place into a large mixing bowl.

Once squash is cooked, let cool for 10 minutes, then gently scrape with the tines of a kitchen fork around the edges of the squash to shred the pulp into spaghetti strands. Put spaghetti into the bowl with the onion and spinach mixture, add pesto sauce, and mix well. Divide between two plates and serve immediately.

Bison Chili with Herbed "Sour Cream"

1 giant pot

For the Herbed "Sour Cream"

1 cup raw sunflower seeds (unroasted and not salted), soaking optional

¼ cup cold water

¼ teaspoon sea salt

1 tablespoon scallion, minced

1 tablespoon cilantro, minced

1 tablespoon raw apple cider vinegar

Juice of 2 lemons

2 tablespoons olive oil

1 yellow onion, diced small

4–5 garlic cloves, minced

¾ teaspoon sea salt, divided

1 teaspoon cumin

½ teaspoon coriander

1 teaspoon smoked paprika

2 ribs celery, diced

2 carrots, diced

2 red bell peppers, diced

4 scallions, chopped, some reserved for garnish

1 can pinto beans, drained and rinsed

1 can diced tomatoes

4 cups vegetable broth

1 pound ground bison

¼ teaspoon black pepper

3–4 cups kale, destemmed and roughly chopped

1 avocado, sliced, for garnish

To make the herbed "sour cream": Cover sunflower seeds with water and soak for 3 hours or overnight. Pour off all water, and place seeds in the blender. Add ¼ cup cold water, sea salt, scallion, cilantro, apple cider vinegar, and lemon juice. Puree for 3–4 minutes or until completely smooth and creamy in consistency. Use in any recipe that calls for sour cream. Refrigerate in an airtight container for up to a week.

Heat a large soup pot with 1 tablespoon olive oil. Once hot, add diced onion, garlic, and ¼ teaspoon sea salt. Sauté for 2–3 minutes until the onions start to sweat. Next add the dry spices and sauté a couple minutes more. Add the celery, carrots, peppers, scallions, pinto beans, diced tomatoes, vegetable broth, and ¼ teaspoon sea salt and bring to a boil. Reduce the heat to low, cover, and cook until the vegetables are soft, about 15 minutes.

In the meantime, heat a skillet with 1 tablespoon olive oil and place the ground bison in there with ¼ teaspoon sea salt and pepper. Sauté bison, breaking apart with your spoon and gently crumbling. Continue to sauté until the bison is almost fully cooked. Next add it to the soup pot along with the kale and stir to combine. The heat from the soup will wilt the kale.

Ladle soup into bowls and top with a dollop of "sour cream." Garnish with sliced avocado and reserved chopped scallions.

Egg Salad

1 serving

2 hard-boiled eggs, diced
1 tablespoon Healthy Mayonnaise (page 179)
¼ cup onion, finely chopped
½ teaspoon fresh dill, minced (optional)
¼ teaspoon sea salt
⅛ teaspoon black pepper

Place all your ingredients in a mixing bowl and, using a fork, break apart eggs and mix everything together.

Chicken Salad

2 servings

- 2 boneless chicken breasts, cubed and baked without skin
- ¼ cup celery, finely minced
- ¼ cup red onion, finely minced
- ¼ cup raw pecans, chopped
- 1 teaspoon fresh parsley, minced
- ¼ cup Healthy Mayonnaise (page 179)
- 2 tablespoons fresh lemon juice
- ½ teaspoon sea salt
- ½ teaspoon black pepper

Combine all ingredients in a mixing bowl, using a fork. Taste for seasoning. Serve on top of a mixed green salad, in a lettuce wrap, on top of avocado halves, or in a brown rice or almond tortilla wrap.

Homemade Chicken Soup

4 servings

- 2 tablespoons olive oil
- 3 cloves garlic, peeled and chopped
- 1 large yellow onion, chopped
- 1 cup carrots, diced
- 1 cup celery, diced (add tops as well for flavor)
- 1 cup kale, chopped, stems removed
- ½ teaspoon fresh thyme, minced
- ½ teaspoon sea salt, divided
- ¼ teaspoon black pepper
- 2 large chicken breasts, including bones and skin
- 6 cups vegetable broth

Heat 1 tablespoon olive oil into a large soup pot over medium flame and add garlic, onion, carrots, celery, kale, thyme, ¼ teaspoon sea salt, and black pepper. Sauté for 4–5 minutes, until vegetables start to soften and become fragrant.

Add chicken breasts, vegetable broth, and 1/4 teaspoon sea salt. Bring to a boil, then cover with a fitted lid, reduce the heat to low, and simmer for 15–20 minutes, stirring occasionally.

Carefully remove chicken breasts from the soup and place in a bowl to cool enough to be handled. Next remove bone from the breasts and chop up chicken. Place the chicken back in the soup with chopped kale and simmer for another 5–10 minutes so that the flavors are blended. Ladle into bowls and serve.

Thai Spiced Lentil Soup

4 servings

- 1 tablespoon coconut oil
- 1 large yellow onion, diced
- 4 cloves garlic, minced
- 1 inch fresh ginger root, minced
- 1 inch fresh turmeric root, minced
- ½ teaspoon sea salt, divided
- ¼ teaspoon ground cinnamon
- ½ teaspoon black pepper
- 1 teaspoon cumin
- 1 cup celery, diced small
- 1 cup carrot, diced small
- 1½ cups split red lentils, washed and picked through for rocks
- 2 teaspoons red curry paste (Thai Kitchen brand)
- 1 14-ounce can coconut milk
- 4 cups filtered water
- 2 cups kale leaves, chopped
- Cilantro for garnish

In a large stock or soup pot, heat coconut oil over medium heat and sauté onion, garlic, ginger, turmeric, ¼ teaspoon sea salt, cinnamon, black pepper, and cumin. Sauté veggies for 3 to 4 minutes. Next add celery and carrot and sauté for 3 minutes more.

Add split red lentils, red curry paste, coconut milk, filtered water, and ¼ teaspoon sea salt and bring to a boil. Cover with a fitted lid and reduce heat to low. Simmer for 10–12 minutes or until the lentils are tender. Finally add chopped kale, give the soup a stir, and cook for 1 minute more. Serve garnished with cilantro.

Baked Salmon over Leafy Greens

2–3 servings

Olive oil or olive oil spray
1 pound fresh or frozen salmon, cut in half
2 tablespoons grass-fed unsalted butter
Zest of 1 lemon
2 tablespoons scallions, minced and divided
⅛ teaspoon sea salt
Pinch black pepper

For the Dressing

3 tablespoons olive oil
1 tablespoon raw apple cider vinegar
Juice of 1 lemon
Pinch sea salt

For the Salad

2 cups spring greens mix

Preheat the oven to 450°F. If salmon is frozen, place in cold water while still in a sealed package until it has thawed (takes about 20–30 minutes).

Line a baking sheet and spray or drizzle with olive oil. Place salmon skin side down and add both tablespoons of butter, lemon zest, 1 tablespoon scallions, sea salt, and pepper. Bake until salmon is cooked through, about 10–15 minutes, depending on the cut of fish.

In the meantime combine the salad dressing ingredients and place 1 cup of leafy greens on each plate. Once fish is done, place on top of the salad, garnish with another sprinkle of scallions, and drizzle with dressing.

Fish Curry

2 servings

- 1 yellow onion, diced
- 1 inch fresh ginger, peeled and minced
- 1 13.5-ounce can coconut milk, unsweetened
- 2 tablespoons fresh lime juice
- 2 teaspoons red or green curry paste (Thai Kitchen brand)
- 1 teaspoon Coconut Aminos
- 4 drops liquid stevia
- 1 stalk lemongrass, cut into quarters
- ¼ teaspoon sea salt
- 1 pound fresh white fish of your choice, cut into chunks
- 2 cups broccoli
- 2 tablespoons cilantro, minced
- 1 cup cooked quinoa or wild rice, for serving (optional)

Combine onion, ginger, coconut milk, lime juice, curry paste, Coconut Aminos, stevia, lemongrass, and sea salt in a large skillet with a fitted lid. Bring to a boil, reduce heat and cover. Simmer on low heat for 5 minutes.

Add fish, give it a quick stir to combine, and cover with the fitted lid. Simmer for 3 minutes more. Next add the chopped broccoli and simmer for 2 more minutes. Carefully remove all pieces of lemongrass, stir in cilantro, and serve on a bed of quinoa or wild rice.

Chicken Stir-Fry

1 serving

- 1 tablespoon coconut oil
- ½ cup yellow onion, thinly sliced
- ¼ teaspoon sea salt, divided
- ½ cup carrot, thinly sliced
- ½ cup broccoli florets, cut into bite-size pieces

½ cup bok choy, chopped
¼ cup water chestnuts
8 ounces boneless, skinless chicken tenders, cooked and cubed
1 tablespoon Coconut Aminos
Juice of 1 lemon
2 tablespoons scallions, white and green, finely minced
2 tablespoons cilantro, finely minced
1 tablespoon raw sesame seeds, dry-fried in a skillet over medium heat until they smell nutty and turn light brown, 2–3 minutes

Place wok or skillet over medium heat, and add the coconut oil. Once oil is warm, add your onions and ⅛ teaspoon sea salt and sauté for 1–2 minutes. Next add carrots, broccoli, and another ⅛ teaspoon sea salt and sauté for 2 minutes more. Next add bok choy, water chestnuts, chicken, and Coconut Aminos and sauté for about 2–3 minutes more, or until vegetables are desired texture. Remove from heat, stir in lemon juice, scallions, cilantro, and sesame seeds, and serve.

Brown Rice Penne with Chicken Sausage and Vegetables

2 servings

8 ounces brown rice penne (cooked according to package instructions)
2 tablespoons olive oil, divided
2 chicken sausage links (peel off pork casings after cooking)
½ red bell pepper, diced
¼ cup red onion, diced
2 garlic cloves, minced
1 teaspoon thyme
½ teaspoon sea salt, divided
1 cup broccoli, chopped
3 Roma tomatoes, diced (optional)
1 cup fresh arugula, washed and finely chopped

Cook brown rice penne in boiling salted water as directed on package. Rinse cooked noodles, place in a large mixing bowl with 1 tablespoon olive oil, and mix in. Set aside.

Broil chicken sausage links until cooked. Peel off pork casings when cooled. Slice links and put aside. In a large saucepan, heat tablespoon olive oil and add bell peppers, onions, garlic, thyme, and ¼ teaspoon sea salt. Sauté for 3 minutes and then add your broccoli and tomatoes, if using, and sauté for 5 minutes more. Add arugula and the remaining ¼ teaspoon sea salt and cook until wilted. Remove from heat, mix in sliced sausage and penne, and serve.

Vegan or Bison Lasagna

Serves 4–6

- 3 tablespoons olive oil, divided
- 2 large sweet potatoes, thinly sliced the long way
- ½ teaspoon sea salt, divided
- ¼ teaspoon pepper
- ½ pound ground beef or bison (optional)
- 1 9-ounce jar tomato sauce, no sugar added
- 2 medium yellow squashes or zucchini, or 1 of each, thinly sliced the long way
- 1 red onion, finely diced
- 6 cloves garlic, minced
- ¼ cup packed fresh basil, minced
- 1 batch sunflower "cheese" (see below)
- 2 cups baby spinach

For the Sunflower "Cheese"

- 1 cup raw sunflower seeds
- 2 tablespoons raw tahini
- 3 tablespoons agar flakes or tapioca starch
- ¼ cup lemon juice
- 1 tablespoon apple cider vinegar
- 1 teaspoon sea salt
- 3–4 garlic cloves

To make the sunflower "cheese": Blend the ingredients until smooth and creamy, adding ¼ cup water at a time until it is thin enough to blend, but still thick enough to spread.

Preheat oven to 350°F. Line a baking sheet with foil or parchment paper. Also oil an 8-by-8-inch baking dish and set aside. Wash sweet potatoes and slice thinly the long way. Place on baking sheet and drizzle with 2 tablespoons olive oil, ⅛ teaspoon sea salt, and pepper. Use your hands to rub oil over all of the pieces. Bake until soft, about 20 minutes.

If using, sauté beef or bison in a medium skillet with ⅛ teaspoon sea salt for about 5 minutes, stirring constantly and breaking into crumbled pieces. Add the tomato sauce and sauté for 2 minutes more. Place in a bowl and set aside.

While the sweet potato is baking, prepare the yellow squash and/or zucchini by slicing very thinly the long way . . . these are your "noodles." Next, sauté onions and garlic in a medium skillet with 1 tablespoon olive oil and a pinch of sea salt for about 3–5 minutes, until they are soft. Place in a glass bowl and set aside.

Prepare your sunflower "cheese" using the recipe above.

Once the sweet potatoes are done, prepare casserole dish by spooning some of your tomato sauce into the bottom (try getting some without the meat), coating baking dish entirely. Add one layer of cooked sweet potato, one layer of zucchini and/or yellow squash, and a sprinkle of your onion and garlic mixture and fresh basil. Next spread a layer of your Sunflower "Cheese," add a layer of spinach, and top with tomato sauce. Repeat these steps, beginning with the sweet potato and finishing with spinach and tomato sauce. If there is sunflower "cheese" left over, dollop a couple drops on top. Sprinkle with sea salt and pepper.

Place the lasagna in the oven on a baking sheet (in case there are drippings), uncovered, and bake for 45 minutes to 1 hour. After an hour, remove lasagna and let it cool for about 30 minutes, or until the "cheese" is set. Serve on a bed of fresh spinach.

Indian Risotto

2 servings

2 tablespoons ghee (clarified butter)
½ cup yellow onion, minced
1 tablespoon jalapeño pepper, minced
1 teaspoon cumin seeds
½ teaspoon ground turmeric
½ teaspoon sea salt, divided
1 cup mung beans, uncooked
1 cup brown basmati rice, rinsed well in 3 changes of water
1 cup cauliflower, chopped
4½ cups filtered water

Heat ghee in a saucepan and add the onions, jalapeño, cumin seeds, turmeric, and ¼ teaspoon sea salt. Cook until cumin seeds begin to darken. Next add mung beans, brown rice, cauliflower and remaining ¼ teaspoon sea salt and stir to combine. Add water and bring to a boil. Cover with a fitted lid, reduce heat to low, and simmer for 40–45 minutes, or until liquid has been absorbed. Taste for seasoning, and serve.

Tuscan Roast Chicken

3–5 servings, depending on size of chicken

Ingredients
1 roasting chicken, 3 pounds or more, thawed
Bay leaves to taste (4 fresh or 2 dry)
½ lemon (with peel)
Sea salt and fresh ground black pepper
5 garlic cloves, halved

Preheat oven to 400°F. Rinse chicken and wipe dry. Fill cavity with bay leaves, lemon, salt, pepper, and a couple of garlic cloves. Salt and pepper chicken on all sides. Tuck remaining garlic clove halves into the hollows of the thighs and wings. Place chicken on a rack in a roasting pan with about 1 inch of water in the bottom to keep drippings from burning. Reduce temperature to 350°F and bake for 15–30 minutes or until legs move easily and juices run clear.

Optional: Make gravy with pan juices, and pour over a gluten-free grain of your choice.

Roast Duckling

4 servings

For the Chef's Salt

½ cup sea salt

½ tablespoon paprika

½ teaspoon black pepper

1 teaspoon white pepper

1 teaspoon celery salt

1 teaspoon garlic salt (not powder)

4 tablespoons butter

4- to 5-pound duckling, completely defrosted

Chef's Salt (see recipe below)

1 parsnip or carrot, chopped

2 stalks celery, chopped

1 yellow onion, chopped

2 garlic cloves, thinly sliced

4 black peppercorns

1 bay leaf

½ teaspoon marjoram

Mix together all ingredients for Chef's Salt. Preheat oven to 300°F. Spread butter in the bottom of a roasting pan that has a tight-fitting lid. Remove neck and giblets from duck cavity and discard. Rinse duck in cold water and rub inside and out with Chef's Salt. Place duck directly on the butter in the roasting pan, breast side down. Place vegetables and garlic inside and around the duckling. Add about 2 inches of water to the pan. Add the peppercorns and bay leaf, and sprinkle marjoram on the duck and in the water. Cover and cook for 2 hours. Carefully remove duckling to a platter and let it cool (if you don't let it cool, it won't turn out right). Split duckling lengthwise by standing it on the neck end and cutting with a sharp knife from the tip of the tail down the center. Quarter if desired. Save leftovers for soup.

Buckwheat Pizza

4 servings

- ¾ cup plus 2 tablespoons buckwheat flour
- ½ cup tapioca flour
- ½ teaspoon sea salt
- ¼ teaspoon baking soda
- ½ teaspoon garlic powder
- ¼ cup plus 2 tablespoons warm water
- 2 tablespoons olive oil, divided
- 1 large egg
- 1 teaspoon raw apple cider vinegar

For the Toppings

- ¼ cup caramelized red onions
- 3 tablespoons minced garlic
- Pinch sea salt
- ½ cup cooked spinach
- 1 batch Parsley Pesto Sauce (see page 179)
- 2 tablespoons sun-dried tomatoes

In a medium bowl, combine buckwheat flour, tapioca flour, sea salt, baking soda, and garlic powder. In a separate bowl whisk together warm water, 1 tablespoon olive oil, egg, and apple cider vinegar, and then pour into the dry ingredients and mix until fully combined. Cover gently with plastic wrap and let set in the fridge for about 30 minutes. In the meantime heat 1 tablespoon of olive oil in a medium skillet over medium heat. Once oil is hot, add the red onion, garlic, and a pinch of sea salt and sauté for 2 minutes. Next add spinach and sauté for 1 minute more. Cover with a fitted lid and turn off the heat, allowing the residual heat to wilt the spinach. Set aside.

Preheat your oven to 375°F and oil your pizza stone generously. Scoop out about half of the dough onto your baking sheet and, using oiled fingers, spread out on the stone ⅛ inch thick. Bake on bottom rack for about 10 minutes. Carefully remove from the oven and top with pesto spread, the onion-spinach mixture you've set aside, and sun-dried tomatoes. Bake for another 10–12 minutes more, or until the crust starts to turn golden brown.

Turkey Soup with Winter Vegetables

4 servings

2 large turkey legs
2 bay leaves
1 teaspoon dried parsley
1 teaspoon dried thyme
1 teaspoon dried rosemary
1 yellow onion, chopped
2 medium carrots, chopped
3 ribs celery, chopped
1 cup parsnip, chopped
1 cup sweet potato, chopped
¼ teaspoon sea salt
⅛ teaspoon black pepper
6 cups filtered water

Place all of your ingredients into a large slow cooker, cover with water, and cook on low for 8–10 hours. Carefully remove the turkey legs, remove the bones, and shred the meat. Place the meat back in the broth. At this point the soup is finished, but you can slow-cook for 1 hour more to marry the flavors. Season to taste and serve.

Ground Turkey Lettuce Wraps

4 servings

2 tablespoons sesame oil, divided
½ red onion, finely diced
½ cup red bell pepper, diced
1-inch piece ginger root, minced
¼ teaspoon sea salt, divided
1 teaspoon dried dill
1 pound ground turkey, dark or white meat
⅛ teaspoon black pepper
1 teaspoon raw apple cider vinegar
1 tablespoon lime juice
2 drops liquid stevia (optional)
2 tablespoons chives, minced
2 tablespoons cilantro, minced
2 tablespoons sunflower seeds
4 large romaine or butter lettuce leaves for the wraps

Heat 1 tablespoon of sesame oil in a nonstick skillet over medium heat. Once the oil is warm, add the red onion, bell pepper, ginger, ⅛ teaspoon sea salt, and dill and sauté for 2–3 minutes, stirring constantly. Place this in a large mixing bowl. In the same skillet, add another tablespoon of sesame oil and over medium heat add the ground turkey and another ⅛ teaspoon of sea salt and black pepper. Sauté this, breaking it into chunks as you go, for about 5–10 minutes, or until the meat is fully cooked.

Add the turkey to the onion mixture and stir to combine. Finish by adding in apple cider vinegar, lime juice, stevia (if using), chives, cilantro, and sunflower seeds and taste for seasoning. Enjoy wrapped in a lettuce wrap.

African-Style Turkey

4 servings

- 2 tablespoons olive oil
- ½ cup yellow onion, finely diced
- 4 garlic cloves, minced
- 1 tablespoon fresh ginger, minced or grated
- 1 tablespoon fresh turmeric, minced or grated
- ½ teaspoon sea salt, divided
- 1 pound ground turkey
- ½ teaspoon crushed red pepper flakes
- ½ teaspoon dried cinnamon
- ½ cup chicken or vegetable broth
- 1 tablespoon fresh lemon juice
- ¼ teaspoon black pepper
- 2 tablespoons fresh mint, minced

Heat a large skillet (with a fitted lid) over medium heat and add olive oil. Add the onion, garlic, ginger, turmeric, and ¼ teaspoon sea salt and sauté for about 2–3 minutes, stirring constantly to prevent burning. Next add ground turkey, crushed red pepper flakes, cinnamon, and the remaining ¼ teaspoon sea salt and sauté for about 2–3 minutes more, continuing to stir constantly and crumble turkey. Add broth and bring to a boil. Reduce to low, cover, and simmer for about 5–8 minutes more, or until turkey is fully cooked. Add in lemon juice, black pepper, and mint and serve over a gluten-free grain of your choosing.

Marinated Tri-Tip Roast

4 servings

1½- to 2-pound tri-tip roast
½ teaspoon sea salt
½ teaspoon cracked black peppercorns
1 tablespoon garlic cloves, minced
1 tablespoon fresh ginger root, grated
1 tablespoon Coconut Aminos
½ tablespoon white pepper
2 tablespoons xylitol

Place tri-tip in a large zip-lock storage bag. In a mixing bowl combine all the remaining ingredients and then pour into the bag over the tri-tip. Seal the bag and place in the refrigerator for at least an hour, or overnight. Place meat in a roasting pan and cover it with remaining marinade from the plastic bag. Roast at 425°F for 30–35 minutes. When the meat is cooked to desired doneness, carve across the grain into thin slices.

Side Dishes

Mashed Faux-tatoes

4 servings

1 large head of cauliflower
¾ cup unsalted chicken stock
2 garlic cloves, minced
1 tablespoon rosemary, finely chopped
½ teaspoon sea salt, divided
1 tablespoon unsalted butter
2 tablespoons fresh chives, minced
Pinch black pepper

Wash cauliflower and cut into pieces. Combine cauliflower, chicken stock, garlic, rosemary, and ¼ teaspoon sea salt in a 2-quart pan. Bring to a boil and reduce heat. Simmer, covered, until cauliflower is tender, about 20 minutes. Remove from heat, but do not drain the liquid. Add butter and let it melt. Puree the mixture in an immersion blender. Add chives, remaining ¼ sea salt to taste, and black pepper. Mix well again and serve.

Mashed Sweet Potato

2 servings

- 2 cups organic sweet potato, skin on, chopped
- ½ cup filtered water
- ½ cup coconut milk
- ¼ teaspoon sea salt
- 1 tablespoon butter
- ½ teaspoon cinnamon

Place chopped sweet potatoes in a medium saucepan with water, coconut milk, and sea salt. Bring the liquid to a boil, then cover and reduce heat to medium. Simmer 10–12 minutes, or until the sweet potato can be easily pierced with a fork. Cooking time will vary depending on the size of your sweet potato pieces. Once sweet potato is tender, remove from the heat. Add butter and cinnamon and, using a fork, mash everything together. Taste for seasoning and add more sea salt if necessary.

Artichoke with Dipping Sauce

1 serving

1 artichoke
1 bay leaf
⅛ teaspoon sea salt
Healthy Mayonnaise for dipping (page 179)

Wash artichoke. Cut off stem to base and stand upright in a large saucepan. Add 2–3 inches of water to the pan. Add the bay leaf and sprinkle sea salt into the water. Cover and simmer over medium heat until the base is tender—about 45 minutes. Add more water if needed. Serve with Healthy Mayonnaise for dipping.

Stir-Fried Asparagus

2 servings

1 tablespoon olive oil
10–12 spears asparagus
¼ teaspoon sea salt
6 garlic cloves, minced
2 tablespoons slivered almonds
1 small pinch red pepper flakes

Heat wok or skillet with olive oil over medium heat. After 1 minute, add asparagus and sea salt and turn heat to high. Stir-fry for 5 minutes or until asparagus is seared, or lightly browned. Add garlic, slivered almonds, and pepper flakes and stir-fry for about 2 more minutes. Serve hot.

Sautéed Spinach

1–2 servings

2 teaspoons olive oil
3 garlic cloves, minced
½ teaspoon sea salt, divided
2 cups packed spinach, washed
Pinch black pepper

Preheat a medium-size skillet over medium heat with olive oil. Add minced garlic and ⅛ teaspoon sea salt and sauté for 1–2 minutes. Next add spinach with ⅛ teaspoon sea salt and pinch of black pepper and stir to combine. Cover with fitted lid and cook for 2–3 minutes, or until spinach is wilted. Serve immediately.

Broccoli with Sesame Seeds

2 servings

1 large head broccoli, cut into small florets
2 tablespoons raw sesame seeds
2 tablespoons olive oil
1 tablespoon lemon zest
⅛ teaspoon sea salt
1 tablespoon fresh lemon juice

Steam broccoli for 7 minutes. Toast sesame seeds in a dry skillet over low heat for 2–3 minutes, stirring constantly. Pour into a large bowl and set aside. In the same skillet add olive oil, broccoli, lemon zest, and sea salt. Sauté for 2–3 minutes and then add to bowl with sesame seeds. Add lemon juice and combine.

Roasted Brussels Sprouts

3–4 servings

4 cups Brussels sprouts, washed
½ cup olive oil, divided
½ teaspoon sea salt, divided
1 tablespoon raw apple cider vinegar
½ cup yellow onion, diced small
2 tablespoons ginger, minced
Pinch black pepper
Juice and zest of 1 lemon
½ cup walnuts, coarsely chopped (optional)

Preheat oven to 350°F. To prepare Brussels sprouts, remove any yellow or brown outer leaves, cut off the ends, and then cut in half. Place on a baking sheet, pour 3 tablespoons olive oil over them, and sprinkle with ¼ teaspoon sea salt. Using your hands, coat all the Brussels sprouts evenly. Place in the oven and bake for about 15 minutes, remove, and add the apple cider vinegar, toss and bake another 5 minutes more, or until you can pierce them with a fork.

In the meantime heat the remaining 1 tablespoon of olive oil in a medium nonstick skillet over medium heat. Once they are warm, add your onion, ginger, and remaining ¼ teaspoon sea salt and a pinch of black pepper. Sauté this for about 3–4 minutes, or until the onion starts to turn translucent. Place into a large mixing bowl. When the Brussels sprouts are done, add them to the bowl with the onion mixture and pour in the lemon juice and zest. Stir to combine. Next add the chopped walnuts, if using. Serve warm.

Kabocha Squash Slices

4 servings

- Coconut or olive oil spray
- 1 kabocha squash, seeds removed, sliced into ⅛- to ¼-inch wedges
- ¼ cup olive or grapeseed oil
- 1 teaspoon sea salt
- 1 tablespoon rosemary, minced
- 1 teaspoon thyme, minced
- ⅛ teaspoon black pepper

Preheat oven to 400°F. Generously spray a baking sheet with coconut or olive oil spray. Place the kabocha squash in a medium mixing bowl. In a small bowl or measuring cup, mix together ¼ cup grapeseed oil, sea salt, rosemary, thyme, and black pepper and pour over squash. Use your hands to make sure squash is coated well. Place squash on the prepared baking sheet and bake for 10 minutes. Remove from the oven and flip the slices over with a spatula. Continue baking for another 5 minutes, or until desired crispness is reached. Remove squash from pan and place on a wire rack to cool slightly before serving.

Sweetened Butternut Squash

4 servings

- 4 cups butternut squash, seeds removed, peeled and cut into ½- to 1-inch cubes
- 2 tablespoons olive oil or grapeseed oil
- ¼ teaspoon sea salt
- ½ teaspoon cinnamon
- ⅛ teaspoon nutmeg
- 4 drops liquid stevia

Preheat oven to 375°F and line baking sheet with parchment paper. Place the cubed squash on baking sheet. In a small mixing bowl combine remaining ingredients and pour mixture over squash. Using your hands, make sure all pieces are covered evenly. Bake for 20 minutes and then carefully remove and stir to rotate and ensure even cooking. Return the squash to the oven and bake another 15–20 minutes, or until you can pierce through squash. Remove from oven and serve warm as a side dish.

Creamy Carrot Cumin Soup

3–4 servings

2 cups carrots, washed and chopped
1 yellow onion, diced
3 garlic cloves
1 teaspoon dried cumin
1 can coconut milk
1 cup filtered water
¼ teaspoon sea salt
½ teaspoon ground nutmeg

Place all ingredients into a saucepan and bring to a boil. Reduce the heat to low, cover with a fitted lid, and simmer until vegetables are soft, about 15 minutes. Transfer to a blender and blend until smooth and creamy. Season to taste and serve.

Southern Greens Mix

2 servings

1 tablespoon olive oil
¼ cup yellow onion, diced small
1 teaspoon garlic, minced
⅛ teaspoon sea salt, divided
2 cups mixed collard greens, chard, and mustard greens, washed, thick lower stems removed, and chopped
1 tablespoon raw apple cider vinegar

Heat skillet. Add olive oil, onion, garlic, and a pinch of sea salt and sauté for 1–2 minutes. Add greens, apple cider vinegar, and another pinch of sea salt. Cover with fitted lid and sauté over low heat until tender. Serve warm.

Cabbage and Leeks

1 large or 2 small servings

1 cup leeks, white and tender green part
1 tablespoon sesame oil
⅜ teaspoon sea salt, divided
2 cups green cabbage, shredded
2 teaspoons raw apple cider vinegar
2 tablespoons fresh lemon juice
1 tablespoon sesame seeds

Trim the leeks, slice in half lengthwise, wash well, and dry. Slice crosswise into small pieces. Heat a medium skillet over medium heat with sesame oil. Once hot add the leeks and ⅛ teaspoon sea salt and sauté for 2–3 minutes. Next add the shredded cabbage, ¼ teaspoon sea salt, and apple cider vinegar and give it a quick stir. Cover with a fitted lid and let sauté for 3–4 minutes. Turn off the heat and stir in the lemon juice and sesame seeds. Serve warm.

Sesame Millet

3–4 servings

1 cup uncooked millet
3 cups vegetable broth
½ teaspoon sea salt, divided
½ cup raw, hulled sesame seeds
2 tablespoons sesame oil
¼ cup green onions, minced

Wash millet and drain and place in a medium saucepan with a fitted lid. Add the vegetable broth and ¼ teaspoon sea salt and bring to a boil. Cover and reduce heat to low and simmer for 25–30 minutes, or until all the liquid has been absorbed. Let stand for 5–10 minutes to increase fluffiness.

While millet is standing put sesame seeds into a frying pan and toast over low flame for 5 minutes, stirring frequently until golden brown. Once seeds are brown, add the millet and sesame oil, green onions, and remaining ¼ teaspoon sea salt. Stir for another 5 minutes. Serve warm as a side dish.

Quinoa Medley

2 servings

1 cup uncooked quinoa
1¼ cup filtered water
1 tablespoon olive oil
¼ cup red bell pepper, finely diced
¼ cup carrot, finely diced
¼ teaspoon sea salt
2 scallions, minced
3 tablespoons parsley, minced
½ cup dry-roasted pecans, finely chopped
¼ cup (or to taste) Italian Vinaigrette Dressing (see recipe, page 176)

To make the quinoa: Soak raw quinoa for 15 minutes, if possible, to remove the saponin coating, which can have a bitter taste. Rinse quinoa thoroughly. In a saucepan, bring to a boil the water and quinoa, and a pinch of sea salt. Cover and simmer for about 20 minutes. Remove from heat and allow to sit for 5 minutes before serving. Fluff with a fork.

In a skillet, heat 1 tablespoon of olive oil and add peppers, carrot, and ¼ teaspoon sea salt. Sauté for 3–4 minutes and add to your cooked quinoa. Add scallions, parsley, and pecans and slowly add dressing to taste.

Nutty Brown Rice

4 servings

- 2 cups brown basmati rice, rinsed well and soaked for 20 minutes in water, if possible
- 3 teaspoons ground cumin
- ¼ teaspoon ground nutmeg
- ½ teaspoon sea salt
- 2 cups filtered water, for cooking
- ½ cup raw walnuts
- ½ cup raw pecans
- 2 tablespoons sesame oil
- 1 tablespoon Coconut Aminos
- 1 tablespoon fresh parsley, minced

In a pan over low heat, lightly toast basmati rice, cumin, nutmeg, and sea salt stirring constantly for 5 minutes. Add 2 cups of water and bring to a boil. Reduce flame, cover, and simmer for 40 minutes. In a separate pan, roast walnuts and pecans over a low flame, stirring frequently until lightly browned. Once rice is finished cooking, turn off heat and wait 5 minutes before removing lid (this helps unstick rice from the bottom of the saucepan). Place the rice in a large serving bowl and add sesame oil, Coconut Aminos, toasted nuts, and fresh parsley.

Millet Tabouli

2 servings

½ cup millet, uncooked
1¼ cup filtered water
¼ teaspoon sea salt, divided
⅓ cup parsley, chopped
⅓ cup scallions, chopped
2 tablespoons fresh mint, minced
2 tablespoons fresh lemon juice
2 tablespoons olive oil
2 garlic cloves, minced

Rinse millet well in a fine mesh strainer. Place it into a small saucepan with 1¼ cups filtered water and ⅛ teaspoon sea salt and bring to a boil. Reduce heat, cover with a fitted lid and simmer for 20 minutes. Turn off the heat and let sit 5 minutes more. Place the rest of the ingredients in a large mixing bowl, add cooked millet and remaining ⅛ teaspoon sea salt, and toss together lightly.

Sweet Potato or Parsnip Fries

2 servings

2 cups white sweet potato or parsnips, sliced like french fries
¼ cup grapeseed oil
1 teaspoon sea salt
½ teaspoon garlic powder, optional

Preheat oven to 400°F and line a baking sheet with foil. Put sliced sweet potatoes (or parsnips) in a bowl. Pour grapeseed oil and ½ teaspoon sea salt over sweet potatoes and mix to make sure oil covers all sides. Lay out fries on a baking sheet and sprinkle with remaining ½ teaspoon sea salt. Bake at 400°F for 20–30 minutes (depending on how big fries are cut), carefully remove pan from the oven and turn fries over to cook on the other side. Bake for 15–20 minutes more or until fries are golden brown. Serve immediately.

Garlic-Rosemary Paleo Bread

Makes 1 loaf

1 cup almond meal
½ cup coconut flour
½ cup ground flax or chia seeds
1 teaspoon sea salt
½ teaspoon baking soda
1 tablespoon fresh rosemary, minced
6–8 cloves garlic, minced
5 eggs
½ cup olive oil
1 tablespoon raw apple cider vinegar

Preheat your oven to 350°F. Grease an 8½-by-4½-inch glass loaf pan. In a bowl sift together the almond meal, coconut flour, ground flax or chia seeds, sea salt, baking soda, rosemary and garlic. In a separate bowl whisk together eggs, olive oil, and apple cider vinegar. Mix the wet ingredients into the dry ingredients until well combined. Pour batter into the greased loaf pan and place on the middle rack in your oven. Bake for about 40–50 minutes, until it is firm to the touch and golden brown on top.

Let cool for about 5–10 minutes before removing from loaf pan. Finish cooling on a rack, or slice.

Note: This bread may be stored in an airtight container in the refrigerator for 5–7 days, or you can slice it and store in the freezer for a month.

Salads

Arugula, Beet, and Walnut Salad

2 servings

4 cups arugula, washed well (discard stems)

¼ cup red onion, thinly sliced

½ cup green apple, thinly sliced

¼ cup beet, shredded

¼ cup raw walnuts (dry roast at 350° in oven for 10 minutes)

Italian Vinaigrette Dressing (see page 176)

Brazil Nut "Cheese" (see page 182)

Assemble all of the ingredients on a large plate. Drizzle with 2 tablespoons of dressing and sprinkle with "cheese."

Butter Lettuce, Hard-Boiled Egg, and Nutty "Parmesan"

2 servings

2 large hard-boiled eggs, cut into wedges

1 teaspoon olive oil

¼ cup red onion, sliced thinly

2 cups butter lettuce leaves

1 small carrot, grated (about ¼ cup)

¼ cup Brazil Nut "Cheese" (see recipe, page 182)

For the Dressing

2 tablespoons extra virgin olive oil

1 tablespoon raw apple cider vinegar

1 tablespoon minced chives

⅛ teaspoon sea salt

Pinch black pepper

To prepare the hard-boiled eggs, place eggs in a small saucepan in single layer. Add cold water to cover eggs by about 1 inch. Heat over high heat just to boiling, then remove from burner and cover the pan with a fitted lid. Let the eggs stand in the hot water for about 12 minutes (about 9 minutes for medium sized eggs and 15 minutes for extra large eggs). Once time is up, drain the hot water and let eggs cool under cold running water or place in a large bowl of ice water. Finally carefully peel eggs and cut into wedges. Set aside.

Now heat a small skillet over medium heat with 1 teaspoon olive oil and add the sliced onion. Sauté onion for 4–5 minutes, or until soft. Set aside. To prepare salad, wash and dry butter lettuce and place on two plates. Top with red onion, carrot, hard-boiled eggs, and a sprinkle of "cheese." Finish by drizzling dressing on each plate.

Marinated Kale Salad

2 servings

- 4 cups black kale, ribs removed, leaves chopped
- 3 tablespoons olive or avocado oil
- Zest and juice of 1 lemon
- 1 tablespoon raw apple cider vinegar
- ½ teaspoon sea salt
- ½ cup tomatoes, diced
- 1 carrot, grated
- ¼ cup red onion, diced
- ½ avocado, diced
- Italian Vinaigrette Dressing (optional; see page 176)

Place kale in a large mixing bowl. In a separate bowl, whisk together oil, lemon juice and zest, apple cider vinegar, and sea salt. Pour the dressing over the kale and massage into the leaves until they are soft. Add tomatoes, carrot, red onion, and avocado to the kale and toss to combine. Add Italian Vinaigrette Dressing to taste, if desired. Taste for seasoning and serve.

Chopped Taco Salad

2 servings

Taco Seasoning

2 teaspoons chili powder

1½ teaspoon smoked paprika

1 teaspoon onion powder

½ teaspoon sea salt

½ teaspoon garlic powder

½ teaspoon cumin

½ teaspoon oregano

½ teaspoon black pepper

1 pinch cayenne pepper

1 pinch red pepper flakes

1 tablespoon olive oil

½ cup red onion, diced small

4 cloves garlic, minced

Pinch sea salt

1 can black beans, drained and rinsed well

2 tablespoons taco seasoning (see below)

½ cup cherry tomatoes, chopped

¼ cup carrot, shredded

2 tablespoons fresh cilantro, minced

2 cups mixed greens

½ avocado, sliced

Juice of 1 lime

Combine ingredients for taco seasoning in a small bowl. Heat a medium skillet with 1 tablespoon of olive oil. Sauté red onion and garlic with a pinch of sea salt for 1–2 minutes. Next add black beans and taco seasoning and sauté for 2–3 minutes more. Add the cherry tomatoes, carrot, and cilantro and pour into a large bowl. Set aside. To serve, divide greens between 2 plates and top each with half the black bean mix and avocado slices. Squeeze the juice of half a lime over the top of each and enjoy.

Cucumber Salad

2 servings

- 2 cups cucumber, diced
- ½ cup cherry tomatoes, diced
- 1 tablespoon red onion, minced
- 1 tablespoon basil, minced
- 1 tablespoon olive oil
- 1 tablespoon lemon juice
- 1 tablespoon lemon zest
- 1 teaspoon raw apple cider vinegar
- Pinch sea salt

Combine cucumber, tomatoes, and red onion in a mixing bowl. In a small bowl or measuring cup, whisk together all the dressing ingredients. Pour over salad mixture and serve.

Avocado Salad

2 servings

- 1 cup avocado, diced
- ½ cup cucumber, diced
- 8–10 black olives (without vinegar), minced
- 1 tablespoon red onion, minced
- 1 tablespoon cilantro, minced
- 2 teaspoons garlic, minced
- 1 tablespoon lime juice
- Pinch sea salt
- Pinch pepper

Combine avocado, cucumber, olives, and red onion in a mixing bowl. In a small bowl or measuring cup, whisk together the remaining ingredients. Pour over salad mixture and serve.

Spinach Salad

2 servings

1 cup packed spinach, washed
¼ cup cucumber, chopped
1 tablespoon carrot, shredded
1 tablespoon olive oil
Pinch sea salt
Pinch black pepper
Brazil Nut "Cheese" topping (optional; see page 182)

Combine the spinach, cucumber, and carrots on a plate. Drizzle with olive oil, sea salt, and pepper. Sprinkle Brazil Nut "Cheese" on top.

Asian Coleslaw

3–4 servings

3 cups cabbage, chopped
1 carrot, grated
¼ cup daikon radish, grated
2 tablespoons green onions, finely chopped
½ teaspoon sea salt
1 green apple, finely sliced
2 tablespoons raw sesame seeds
Pinch black pepper
Pinch red pepper flakes (optional)

For the Dressing

2 tablespoons sesame oil
1 tablespoon raw apple cider vinegar
1 tablespoon fresh lime juice
2 drops liquid stevia
Pinch sea salt

Place the cabbage, carrot, daikon, and green onions in a large mixing bowl and sprinkle with sea salt. Using your hands, massage the sea salt into the mixture to break it down. You will notice the cabbage start to get softer. Next add the green apple, sesame seeds, black pepper, and red pepper flakes, if using. In a small mixing bowl whisk together the coleslaw dressing ingredients and then pour over your coleslaw. Mix everything together.

Sauces, Dressings, and Dips

Italian Vinaigrette Dressing

Makes about 1 cup

¾ cup olive oil
¼ cup raw, unfiltered apple cider vinegar
1 rosemary sprig, chopped
1 cup fresh basil leaves, chopped
3 garlic cloves, peeled and mashed
1 teaspoon dry mustard (optional)
5 drops liquid stevia

Put all ingredients in a lidded jar and shake well. Store in the refrigerator in an airtight glass jar for up to 2 weeks.

Cumin Vinaigrette

Makes about ¾ cup

½ cup olive oil
1 teaspoon Eden Foods Organic Yellow (or Brown) Mustard
2 tablespoons fresh lemon juice
½ teaspoon ground cumin
½ teaspoon minced garlic
2 tablespoons raw apple cider vinegar
¼ teaspoon sea salt

Put all ingredients in a lidded jar and shake well. Store in the refrigerator in an airtight glass jar for up to 2 weeks.

Ranch Dressing

Makes 2 cups

- 1 cup raw hempseeds
- ½ cup olive oil
- ¼ cup fresh lemon juice
- ¼ cup filtered water, more if necessary
- 2 tablespoons Coconut Aminos
- 3 garlic cloves
- 1–2 tablespoons jalapeño pepper, seeded and chopped (optional)
- ½ teaspoon sea salt
- ⅛ teaspoon black pepper
- 2 tablespoons fresh dill, minced
- 2 tablespoons chives, minced

Place all ingredients (except for dill and chives) into a blender and blend starting at a low speed and gradually increase, scraping down the sides as necessary. Blend until smooth and creamy, adding more filtered water 1 tablespoon at a time if necessary. Add fresh herbs and blend again until they are incorporated. Overblending at this point will cause the mixture to turn green. Enjoy with sliced vegetables, gluten-free crackers, or as a salad dressing. Store in the refrigerator in an airtight glass jar for up to 2 weeks.

Ginger-Wasabi Dressing

Makes about 1 cup

½ cup olive oil
2 tablespoons ginger, freshly grated
1 tablespoon fresh horseradish root, grated
2 tablespoons raw apple cider vinegar
1 teaspoon sea salt

Place all ingredients into a blender and blend for 2–3 minutes. Use this dressing over salads or fish. Store in the refrigerator in an airtight glass jar for up to 2 weeks.

Tahini Dressing

Makes ½ cup

Ingredients
¼ cup raw tahini butter (Artisana), unsalted
1 tablespoon raw apple cider vinegar
2 tablespoons filtered water
2 tablespoons fresh lemon juice
4 drops liquid stevia
¼ teaspoon sea salt
Pinch black pepper

Place all ingredients into a mixing bowl and whisk with a fork to combine. This dressing is great paired with sliced raw vegetables or served as a dip with gluten-free crackers. Store in the refrigerator in an airtight glass jar for up to 1 week.

Healthy Mayonnaise

Makes 1 cup

- 1 egg
- 1 teaspoon Eden Foods Organic Yellow (or Brown) Mustard
- 1 tablespoon raw apple cider vinegar or fresh lemon juice
- ¼ teaspoon sea salt
- ¾ cup grapeseed oil or sunflower seed oil

Put the egg, mustard, vinegar or lemon juice, and sea salt in a blender or food processor. Blend until smooth. Slowly add in oil while blending on low until smooth and creamy. Store in the refrigerator in an airtight glass jar for up to 2 weeks.

Parsley Pesto Sauce

Makes 1 to 1½ cups

- 2 cups loosely packed fresh Italian parsley, large stems removed
- ½ cup raw macadamia or pine nuts
- ¼ cup olive oil
- 2 garlic cloves, minced
- 1 tablespoon lemon juice
- ½ teaspoon sea salt
- Pinch black pepper

Strip parsley leaves from the stems. Finely chop leaves and place in a blender or food processor and pulse a couple times. Toast nuts in a skillet over medium heat until you smell a nutty flavor and they turn light brown, 2–3 minutes. Remove the nuts from the heat and allow to cool. Add the toasted nuts, olive oil, garlic, lemon juice, sea salt, and black pepper to the food processor and pulse until combined.

You may need to stop several times to scrape down the edges. Taste for seasoning. Serve as a dip with raw or roasted vegetables, or drizzle over gluten-free pasta or eggs. Store in the refrigerator in an airtight glass jar for up to 1 week.

No-Cheese Pesto

Makes about 2 cups

- 3 cups fresh basil
- ¾ cup olive oil
- 1 teaspoon sea salt
- 4 garlic cloves, peeled
- ½ cup dry-roasted pine nuts
- 2 tablespoons fresh lemon juice

Blend all ingredients in blender. Serve the pesto over vegetables or brown rice pasta. Store in the refrigerator in an airtight glass jar for up to 1 week.

Herbed "Sour Cream"

Makes about 1 cup

- 1 cup raw sunflower seeds (unroasted and not salted)
- ¼ cup water
- ¼ teaspoon sea salt
- 1 tablespoon scallion, minced
- 1 tablespoon cilantro, minced
- 1 tablespoon raw apple cider vinegar
- Juice of 2 lemons

Cover sunflower seeds with water and soak for a few hours, or overnight. Pour off all the water and place seeds in a blender. Add ¼ cup cold water, sea salt, scallions, cilantro, apple cider vinegar, and lemon juice. Puree for 3–4 minutes or until completely smooth and creamy in consistency. Use in any recipe that calls for sour cream. Refrigerate in an airtight container for up to 1 week.

Olive Tapenade

Makes about ½ cup

½ cup black olives, pitted and chopped
2 tablespoons fresh lemon juice
1 teaspoon raw apple cider vinegar
1 tablespoon olive oil
⅛ teaspoon sea salt
1 tablespoon parsley, minced
1 tablespoon scallion, minced
¼ cup dry-roasted pine nuts, finely chopped

Hand mix all ingredients.Serve with gluten-free crackers or use as a sauce for fish dishes. Store in the refrigerator in an airtight glass jar for up to 1 week.

Garlic and Cilantro Marinade

Makes about ½ cup

¼ cup lime juice
4 garlic cloves, small, minced
2 tablespoons cilantro, minced
1 teaspoon raw apple cider vinegar
1 teaspoon Coconut Aminos
6 drops liquid stevia
¼ cup olive oil
⅛ teaspoon sea salt
Pinch red pepper flakes (optional)

Place all ingredients into a mixing bowl and use a fork to combine. Marinade can be used over chicken or fish dishes or used for a stir-fry. Store in the refrigerator in an airtight glass jar for up to 2 weeks.

Brazil Nut "Cheese"

Makes 1 cup

1 cup raw Brazil nuts (do not soak)
4–6 cloves garlic
1 tablespoon olive oil
1 teaspoon sea salt

Rinse the Brazil nuts in a colander and set aside. Place the garlic in a food processor and pulse for a couple of seconds. Add the Brazil nuts, olive oil, and sea salt, and pulse until the nuts crumble and get sticky. Store in an airtight container in the refrigerator or freezer.

If you cannot handle eating raw garlic, try blanching the garlic (put cloves in boiling water for 5 minutes). This will slightly alter the taste of the "cheese." Store in the refrigerator in an airtight glass jar for up to 2 weeks or in the freezer for up to one month.

Guacamole

Makes about 1 cup

1 medium-size ripe avocado, peeled and pitted
Juice of 1 lime
1 teaspoon onion, finely chopped
⅛ teaspoon sea salt
Pinch black pepper
Fresh cilantro, chopped (optional)

In a mixing bowl, mash the avocado and then stir in remaining ingredients until combined; taste and adjust seasoning as desired. Enjoy as a dip for raw vegetables, with gluten-free crackers, or on top of a burger. Store in the refrigerator in an airtight glass jar for up to 2 days.

Salsa

Makes about 2 cups

1 cup tomatoes, diced
2 tablespoons red onion, finely minced
1 tablespoon olive oil
1 tablespoon fresh lemon juice
1 tablespoon jalapeño pepper, minced
⅛ teaspoon sea salt
Pinch black pepper

Place all ingredients in a small mixing bowl and stir to combine. Serve with turkey lettuce wraps or gluten-free crackers. Store in the refrigerator in an airtight glass jar for up to 3 days.

Homemade Ketchup

Makes about ½ cup

¼ cup tomato paste (canned)
2 tablespoon filtered water
1 tablespoon raw apple cider vinegar
1 tablespoon Coconut Aminos
4 drops liquid stevia
¼ teaspoon sea salt
¼ teaspoon black pepper
3–4 dashes hot sauce (optional; for brands, see page 203)

Combine all ingredients in a bowl and whisk together with a fork. Store in the refrigerator in an airtight glass jar for up to 2 weeks.

Almond Butter Dipping Sauce

Makes about 1½ cups

1 cup dry-roasted almond butter, unsalted
¼ cup filtered water
1 tablespoon fresh lemon juice
1 teaspoon raw apple cider vinegar
3 drops liquid stevia
⅛ teaspoon sea salt

Place all ingredients in a mixing bowl and using a fork mix until desired consistency is reached. Store in the refrigerator in an airtight glass jar for up to 2 weeks.

Macadamia Cream Sauce

Makes about 1 cup

15 raw macadamia nuts, soaking optional (4–8 hours)
1/8 teaspoon sea salt
1 tablespoon fresh lemon juice
1 drop liquid stevia
1 garlic clove (optional)

Blend all ingredients in blender. Add more lemon juice if needed for desired consistency. Store in the refrigerator in an airtight glass jar for up to 2 weeks.

Desserts and Snacks

Baked Cinnamon Apple

2 servings

2 medium Granny Smith or Pippin apples
2 tablespoons unsalted butter, softened
½ teaspoon ground cinnamon
Pinch sea salt
Pinch nutmeg (optional)

Remove apple core to about ½ inch from the bottom of the apple. Make the hole about ¾ to 1 inch wide. Blend butter, cinnamon, sea salt, and nutmeg if using. Spoon it into cavity of apples. Place apple in a buttered baking dish with about ¼ inch of water, cover with foil, and bake at 350°F for about 15 minutes. Remove foil and bake about 5 minutes more or until tender. Remove from oven and let cool slightly. Serve warm.

Carrot Muffins

Makes 12 muffins

- Silicone muffin tin or muffin tin liners
- Coconut or olive oil spray
- 1 tablespoon chia seeds
- ¾ cup warm water
- 2 teaspoons raw apple cider vinegar
- 2 tablespoons grapeseed oil
- 1 teaspoon vanilla extract
- 1 tablespoon fresh lemon juice
- ¾ cup almond meal
- 1 cup sweet sorghum flour
- ¼ cup xylitol
- 1 teaspoon baking soda
- 1 teaspoon baking powder
- 1 teaspoon cinnamon
- ¼ teaspoon sea salt
- 1½ cups carrot, shredded
- ½ cup raw walnuts, chopped

Preheat oven to 350°F. Grease muffin tin with coconut or olive oil spray or use muffin tin liners. Place the chia seeds, water, apple cider vinegar, grapeseed oil, vanilla, and lemon juice in a blender and let sit for about 5 minutes so that the chia seeds plump up.

In a large bowl, place the almond meal, sorghum flour, xylitol, baking soda, baking powder, cinnamon, and sea salt and whisk well to evenly combine. After chia seed mixture has been in the blender for 5 minutes, blend for 1–2 minutes. Pour mixture into the bowl of dry ingredients and mix well. Stir in the shredded carrots and chopped walnuts. Using a spoon or ice cream scoop, drop the batter into the muffin tin or liners, filling them ¾ full. Tap muffin tin gently on the counter to pop any air bubbles. Bake for about 25 minutes (15–20 minutes if using a mini muffin tin). Remove from oven and place muffin tin on a cooling rack. Allow the muffins to cool in the pan for about five minutes to set, then carefully remove muffins from the tin and continue to cool on cooling rack. Store leftover muffins in an airtight container in the refrigerator for up to 1 week.

Baked Apple Crumble

6–8 servings

3–4 green apples, cut into ¼ inch slices
2 tablespoons xylitol
10 drops liquid stevia
1 heaping tablespoon arrowroot
1 teaspoon ground cinnamon
¼ teaspoon ground nutmeg
¼ cup filtered water
Juice of one lemon
1 tablespoon vanilla extract
Pinch sea salt

For the Crumble

1 cup quick cooking oats, gluten-free
½ cup raw sunflower seeds or slivered almonds
¼ cup coconut flour
¼ cup almond meal
¼ cup xylitol
½ teaspoon baking powder
¼ teaspoon baking soda
¼ teaspoon sea salt
½ cup butter, melted

Preheat the oven to 350°F. Place the apples in an oiled pie dish. In a small bowl whisk together xylitol, stevia, arrowroot, cinnamon, nutmeg, water, lemon juice, vanilla, and sea salt and pour over the apples.

In a separate bowl combine the oats, sunflower seeds, coconut flour, almond meal, xylitol, baking powder, baking soda, and sea salt. Melt the butter in a small saucepan and pour over the mixture. Crumble this evenly over the apples.

Cover with foil and bake for 30–35 minutes, or until the apples are tender. Remove the foil for the last 5–10 minutes of baking to brown the crumble. Serve warm.

Gluten-Free Crepes

Makes 3–4 crepes

¼ cup arrowroot or tapioca flour
1 tablespoon coconut flour
¼ teaspoon baking soda
¼ teaspoon baking powder
½ teaspoon cinnamon
⅛ teaspoon sea salt
2 eggs
1 tablespoon grapeseed oil
1 teaspoon raw apple cider vinegar
½ teaspoon vanilla extract
3 drops liquid stevia
Coconut or olive oil spray

In a small bowl whisk together arrowroot or tapioca flour, coconut flour, baking soda, baking powder, cinnamon, and sea salt. In a separate bowl whisk together eggs, grapeseed oil, apple cider vinegar, vanilla, and stevia.

Combine dry ingredients with wet and whisk together to remove any lumps. Heat a nonstick skillet over medium heat and spray generously with oil spray. When hot, spoon ¼ cup of batter onto the skillet and slightly rotate it around in a circle to help distribute the batter. Let cook for 1 minute, then flip with spatula and cook the other side for about 30 seconds more. Remove crepe from heat and spread with nut butter or desired filling. Serve warm.

Baked Berries

4 servings

1 16-ounce bag organic frozen berries
3 tablespoons filtered water, at room temperature
1 tablespoon tapioca or arrowroot flour
1 teaspoon vanilla extract
Pinch sea salt
3 drops liquid stevia

Preheat oven to 350°F. Place berries in an 8-by-8-inch baking dish. In a small bowl combine water, flour, vanilla, sea salt, and stevia. Pour over the berries and mix. Cover with foil and bake for about 20–25 minutes, or until berries are cooked and liquid has thickened.

Ginger Spiced Cookies

9 large or 12 small cookies

Coconut oil spray
½ cup almond butter
½ cup shredded unsweetened coconut
¼ cup xylitol
1 teaspoon ginger powder
1 teaspoon cinnamon
1 egg
¼ teaspoon sea salt

Preheat oven to 350°F. Line a baking sheet with parchment paper and spray with coconut oil spray. Put remaining ingredients in a food processor and blend until fully combined. Place 1–2 tablespoons of batter at a time onto a baking sheet, depending on size of cookie you are making. Press batter down with a fork to flatten, and bake for 15–18 minutes, or until cookies turn golden brown. Let cool on a cooling rack. Store in an airtight container in the refrigerator for up to 2 weeks.

Paleo Cacao Nib Cookies

Makes 12 cookies

Coconut oil spray
1 cup almond flour
¼ cup tapioca flour
¼ cup xylitol
1 tablespoon shredded unsweetened coconut
½ teaspoon ground cinnamon
½ teaspoon baking soda
⅛ teaspoon sea salt
2 tablespoons coconut oil
1 egg
½ tablespoon vanilla extract
⅓ cup cacao nibs

Preheat oven to 350°F. Line a baking sheet with parchment paper and spray with coconut oil spray. In a medium bowl, whisk together almond flour, tapioca flour, xylitol, shredded coconut, cinnamon, baking soda, and sea salt, removing any lumps.

In a separate bowl combine coconut oil, egg, and vanilla. Mix wet ingredients into the dry and then add in the cacao nibs.

Using a mini ice cream scoop, scoop 1 tablespoon at a time onto a prepared baking sheet, leaving about 1 inch between each spoonful of batter. After all the batter is placed on the baking sheet, flatten each one slightly with the palm of your hand. Bake for 8–10 minutes, or until they just start to turn brown. Remove baking sheet from oven and carefully transfer to a rack to cool completely. Store in an airtight container in refrigerator for up to 2 weeks.

Chocolate Avocado Pudding

2 servings

- 1 large ripe avocado, about 1 cup
- ¼ cup unsweetened cocoa powder
- ¼ cup coconut cream
- 2 tablespoons xylitol
- 5 drops liquid stevia
- 1 teaspoon vanilla extract
- Pinch sea salt
- 1–2 tablespoons nondairy milk, if necessary, to make creamy
- Unsweetened shredded coconut, for garnish

Place all the ingredients except for the shredded coconut into a food processor and blend until smooth and creamy, stopping occasionally to scrape down the sides. If mixture is too thick, add nondairy milk 1 tablespoon at a time until the desired consistency is reached. Serve with a sprinkle of unsweetened shredded coconut.

Spicy Almonds, Walnuts, or Pecans

4–6 servings

- 2 cups raw almonds, walnuts, or pecans
- 1 tablespoon unsalted grass-fed butter, melted
- 2 dashes cayenne pepper
- 4 drops liquid stevia
- ¼ teaspoon sea salt

Preheat oven to 300°F. Line a baking sheet with parchment paper. Place nuts into a mixing bowl. In a separate dish stir together your butter, cayenne pepper, stevia, and sea salt. Pour into the nut mixture and stir to combine. Spread mixture onto your prepared baking sheet and bake for 10 minutes, or until fragrant and golden brown.

Kale Chips

2 servings

1 bunch kale, stems removed
1 tablespoon olive oil
¼ teaspoon sea salt
Pinch black pepper
Other spices as desired

Preheat oven to 300°F. Line a baking sheet with parchment paper. Remove stems from kale. Wash kale leaves, dry, cut into pieces and place in a mixing bowl with olive oil, sea salt, black pepper, and other spices, if using. Use your hands to gently massage the ingredients into the kale. Bake until edges start to slightly brown, about 10–15 minutes. Cool before serving.

Sorghum Popcorn

1 serving

¼ cup Tru-Pop Popping Sorghum
1 tablespoon olive oil
⅛ teaspoon sea salt

Add a few grains to a tall-sided pot and heat over medium heat. When the first grains pop, add the rest of the sorghum and stir very slowly with a wooden spoon. When popping begins, cover and turn heat down slightly. Continue to move the grains around by gently shaking the pot handle. When popping slows, remove from heat. Drizzle with olive oil and sprinkle with sea salt or other seasonings of your desire. About 60 to 70 percent of the grains will pop, but the whole batch is edible.

Beverages

Raspberry Lemonade

2 servings

¼ cup fresh raspberries
¼ cup freshly squeezed lemon juice
2 cups filtered water
4 drops liquid stevia
1 tablespoon xylitol

Place all the ingredients in a blender and blend until smooth. Serve over ice if desired.

Hot or Cold Cocoa/Cacao Milk

1 serving

1 cup unsweetened almond milk (plain)
½ teaspoon vanilla extract (alcohol-free)
2 tablespoons raw cacao powder or unsweetened cocoa powder
4 drops liquid stevia
1 tablespoon xylitol
Pinch sea salt

Place all ingredients in a blender and give a quick blend to combine. Pour into a small saucepan and heat over low heat for 2–3 minutes or until warm. If desired cold, just pour from your blender into a cup.

Hibiscus-Mint Cooler (Sun Tea)

6–8 servings

8 cups filtered water
½ cup hibiscus flowers
½ cup fresh mint leaves

Put hibiscus flowers, mint leaves, and water in glass jar and set outside in direct sunlight to make sun tea. Bring inside after an hour or two. Strain, and chill in refrigerator. Serve over ice.

Yerba Mate Latte

Makes 1 large cup

1½ cups filtered water
½ cup almond or hemp milk, unsweetened
1 teaspoon coconut oil
1 tablespoon yerba mate powder
¼ teaspoon cinnamon
2–3 drops liquid stevia (optional)

Bring the water to a boil. Meanwhile, place the almond or hemp milk, coconut oil, yerba mate powder, and cinnamon into a blender. Add boiling water and cover tightly. Starting on low speed, begin to blend, gradually increasing to high. Blend for 30–45 seconds, or until mixture starts to look frothy. Pour into your favorite coffee mug.

Citrus Soda

1 serving

1 cup sparkling mineral water, such as Gerolsteiner
1 wedge of fresh lemon or lime
3–4 drops liquid stevia

Place all the ingredients in a glass and serve.

Ginger Ale

2 servings

¾ cup ginger root, peeled and chopped
4 cups filtered water
2 tablespoons alcohol-free vanilla extract
1 tablespoon alcohol-free lemon extract
10 or more drops liquid stevia
Sparkling mineral water, such as Gerolsteiner

Place chopped ginger and water in a medium saucepan and bring to a rapid boil over medium-high heat. Cover with a fitted lid and reduce heat to medium-low. Simmer for about 10–15 minutes. Carefully strain the liquid into a jar and discard the ginger. Stir in vanilla, lemon, and stevia and place in the refrigerator to cool. Add sparkling mineral water to desired concentration when serving.

Kale-Ginger Cleanser

1 serving

- 1 bunch kale, center stems removed
- 1-inch piece fresh ginger root
- 1 small bunch parsley (4–5 stems), with stems, or small bunch watercress
- ½ green apple
- 1 lemon
- 3 or more drops liquid stevia (optional)

Place first five ingredients in a vegetable juice extractor. Add stevia if using.

Vegetable Alkalizer Juice

1 serving

- 3 stalks celery
- ½ small carrot
- ½ Granny Smith apple (no seeds)
- 1 medium cucumber
- 2 cups raw spinach, watercress, chard, dark green lettuce, and/or black kale,* dandelion greens, cilantro and/or parsley
- 1 small garlic clove (optional)
- 1-inch slice of turmeric root, and/or 1-inch slice of ginger root (optional)
- ½ fresh lemon

Place all the ingredients in a vegetable juice extractor. Drink juice immediately on an empty stomach either an hour before or 2–3 hours after a meal.

Note: Limit black kale to two or three times a week, due to its potential thyroid-inhibiting effect.

Lemon-Poppyseed Shake

1 serving

1 cup unsweetened coconut, almond, or hemp milk
½ cup ice cubes
1 tablespoon poppyseeds
1 tablespoon flaxseed oil
1 tablespoon fresh lemon juice
1 scoop egg-white protein powder
2 tablespoons nut butter (almond or macadamia)

Place all the ingredients in a blender and blend until smooth.

Blueberry–Pumpkin Seed Shake

1 serving

1 cup unsweetened coconut milk (not low-fat), almond milk, or hemp milk
½ cup fresh or frozen blueberries
1 tablespoon flaxseed oil
1 scoop unflavored pumpkin-seed protein powder (Pure Goodness)
½ teaspoon cinnamon
5–10 drops liquid stevia

Place all the ingredients in a blender and blend until smooth and creamy.

Protein Smoothie

1 serving

- 2 cups unsweetened coconut milk
- 1 scoop egg-white protein powder
- 1 cup fresh strawberries, washed and stems removed
- 1 cup raw spinach
- ¼ cup avocado, chopped
- 2 tablespoons chia seeds
- 1 tablespoon xylitol or 5–6 drops liquid stevia

Place all ingredients in a blender and blend until smooth and creamy.

Almond Milk

About 6 cups

- 1 cup blanched almonds, soaked in filtered water 4–6 hours overnight
- 6 cups filtered water
- ⅛ teaspoon sea salt
- 1 teaspoon alcohol-free vanilla extract
- 5–6 drops liquid stevia

Start by draining and rinsing soaked almonds in a fine mesh strainer. Place all ingredients in a blender and blend for 2–3 minutes. Strain through a very fine mesh strainer (or through cheesecloth) into a large jar with a fitted lid. Taste for seasoning. A batch will stay good in the refrigerator for 4–5 days.

Herbal Teas

There are various herbal teas to choose from—lavender, mint, rooibos, chamomile, hibiscus, and dandelion root, for instance. I prefer no caffeine while doing your 90-day program, with the exception of white tea, which although it contains small amounts of caffeine will not disrupt the endocrine system and is an excellent blood cleanser, removing toxins from the body. If your body tolerates caffeine, you can drink one or two cups a day. Add stevia, lo han, or xylitol to sweeten if desired.

Recommended Products

Many of the recipes in this chapter include ingredients that can usually be found in your local health food store or ordered online. Buying some of these products and keeping them on hand will give you a head start and help make your daily food choices easier. If your store does not carry an item listed below, let them know you are a regular customer and ask them to special-order it for you, or go on the Internet and order directly from the company or affiliated sites—vitacost.com, iherb.com, thrivemarket.com, and amazon.com, among others—that sell those products.

Bread	**Brand**
Almond flour mix gluten-free artisan bread	Simple Mills
Breads (yeast-, gluten-, dairy-, and sugar-free)	
Brown rice or black rice tortillas	Food for Life
Original and turmeric coconut wraps	Nuco
Broth	**Brand**
Organic free-range chicken broth, organic vegetable broth	Imagine, Pacific

Butter	Brand
Goat's-milk butter	Liberté
Organic butter (unsalted)	Horizon

Cereal, Cold	Brand
Qi'a Superfood–chia, buckwheat, and hemp cereal (original flavor)	Nature's Path
Simple granola	Go Raw
Sprouted cinnamon cereal	Lydia's Organics

Cereal, Hot	Brand
Amaranth, brown rice, teff, oatmeal (gluten-free, after 3 months)	Bob's Red Mill
Brown rice cream	Erewhon
Cream of buckwheat	Pocono
Quinoa flakes	Ancient Harvest

Condiments	Brand
Coconut butter	Artisana
Garlic spreads (various flavors)	Majestic Garlic
Guacamole	Trader Joe's, 365 (Whole Foods)
Liquid aminos (unfermented soy sauce and soy-free seasoning)	Bragg, Coconut Secret
Mustard (with apple cider vinegar only)	Trader Joe's, 365 (Whole Foods), Eden Foods Organic Yellow/Brown Mustard
Organic Sea Kelp Delight Seasoning	Bragg
Pestos, dairy-free (spicy and mild)	Basiltops
Sea salt, Celtic sea salt	HimalaSalt, Grain & Salt Society, Real Salt

Oil	Brand
Coconut, flaxseed, grapeseed, olive oils that are cold-pressed or expeller-pressed	Spectrum

Crackers	Brand
Almond crackers (fine-ground, rosemary sea salt, sundried tomato, and basil)	Simple Mills
Brown rice cakes	Lundberg
Brown rice crackers	Hol-Grain Crackers
Cracked pepper and sea salt, Mediterranean, and Tuscan	Crackerz Jilz Gluten Free
Flax and herb crackers (read ingredients)	Raw Makery
Flax crackers (raw crisps and crusts)	Mauk Family Farms
Garden herb, pesto, and tomato basil	Two Moms in the Raw
Hot 'n Spicy Jalapeño Crackers, Super Seed Crackers	Mary's Gone Crackers
Pizza Flax Snax, Sunflower Flax Snax, Spicy Flax Snax, Simple Flax Snax	Go Raw
Pretzels: chipotle tomato, everything	Mary's Gone Crackers
Various crackers (read ingredients)	Awesome Foods

Drinks	Brand
Apple cider vinegar all-natural drinks (Ginger Spice, Limeade, Sweet Stevia)	Bragg
Lemon Love Water	Suja
Mineral water, sparkling	Gerolsteiner
Smart Water	Glaceau

Whole Grains and Flours	Brand
Brown rice	Lundberg
Buckwheat, millet, sorghum, and teff flours (organic)	Arrowhead Mills
Gluten-free grains, flours, wild rice	Bob's Red Mill

Gluten-free pizza dough mix	Simple Mills
Pancake and baking mix, almond meal flour, sweet rice flour, and brown rice flour	Authentic Foods
Quinoa flour (organic)	Ancient Harvest
Waffle and pancake mix, sugar-free muffin mix, Perfect Flour Blend, pizza crust mix	Namaste Foods

Meats, Luncheon*	**Brand**
Herb-roasted turkey, peppered roasted turkey, naturally oven-roasted turkey	Diestel Turkey Ranch
Organic roasted turkey breast, herb turkey breast	Applegate Farms
Oven-roasted turkey (no salt), uncured turkey salami (in deli case)	Whole Foods Market

Note: High in sodium; use small amounts.

Milk Substitutes*	**Brand**
Almond & Cashew Cream, unsweetened (after 3 months)	MimicCreme
Almond milk, coconut milk	365 (Whole Foods)
Almond milk, original and vanilla, unsweetened	Blue Diamond Almond Breeze
Coconut milk, unsweetened	So Delicious
Hemp milk, original, unsweetened	Tempt (Living Harvest)
Organic almond milk, original and vanilla, unsweetened	Pacific Natural Foods
Organic coconut cream, organic coconut milk	Native Forest
Organic coconut milk, unsweetened	Asian Creations–Thai Kitchen

Note: Read the labels, as some of these companies make sweetened and unsweetened varieties with the same name.

Nuts and Seeds, Nut and Seed Butters	**Brand**
Almond butter, sunflower-seed butter	MaraNatha
Coconut butter	Artisana
Pumpkin-seed butter, organic	Jarrow Formulas

Raw nuts, raw or dry-roasted almond butter, macadamia nut butter	Trader Joe's
Raw nuts and nut butters	Whole Foods
Sesame tahini, organic	Arrowhead Mills
Sprouted pumpkin seeds, sunflower seeds, spicy seed mix, simple seed mix	Go Raw
Tahini, organic	Once Again

Pasta	Brand
Brown rice pasta	Lundberg, Trader Joe's
Brown rice pasta, quinoa pasta	Andean Dream
Penne, spaghetti, fettuccine, elbows, etc.	Rizopia Organic
Tinkyada kelp noodles	Sea Tangle Noodle Company

Protein Powders	Brand
Amazing Meal Vanilla Chai Infusion	Amazing Meal
Egg-white protein powder	NOW Foods, MRM
Hemp protein powder, unsweetened	Tempt (Living Harvest)
Instant Whites egg-white protein–plain	Gifted Earth Originals
Protein Energizer Vanilla Shake	Rainbow Light
Pumpkin-seed protein	Pure Goodness (unflavored)
Rice protein, plain or vanilla	NutriBiotic
Rice protein powder: Vanilla Blast, Original, or Chocolate Power (after 2 months)	Growing Naturals

Salsa	Brand
African hot sauces	Brother Bru-Bru's
Habanero salsa	Frontera
Mild or hot salsa	Green Mountain Gringo 365 (Whole Foods)
Salsa	Tacupeto

Snacks/Treats	Brand
Kale chips	Brad's Raw Foods, Alive & Radiant Foods
Nutty Nibbles (sugar-free varieties)	Nut Just a Cookie
Rox Chox (cacao with birch xylitol)	Rox Chox
Steve's Original Paleo Stix (grass-fed beef sticks)	Steve's PaleoGoods
Tru-Pop Popping Sorghum	Just Poppin

Sweeteners	Brand
Chicory root	Just Like Sugar
Lo Han Sweet	Jarrow Formulas
Stevia, liquid and powdered, various flavors	Sweet Leaf, Kal (best tasting)
SweetFiber (inulin fiber, lo han kuo)	Purpose Foods
Xylitol powder (Ultimate Sweetener, Xyla)	Ultimate Life, Xylitol USA

Vinegar*	Brand
Apple cider vinegar, raw and unfiltered	Bragg, Spectrum

Note: Always keep refrigerated.

WHEAT ALTERNATIVES

The following list gives you an idea of the many ways you can enjoy grains and grain substitutes without using wheat, as well as the different forms in which these foods can be found.

Alternative	Available As
Almonds	Flour, meal, almond butter
Amaranth	Flour
Buckwheat	Flour, noodles, whole groats
Chestnut	Flour

Coconut	Flour
Hazelnuts	Flour
Kelp	Noodles
Legumes*	Flours (black bean, fava bean, garbanzo bean, mung bean, pinto bean, red and green lentil, white bean)
Millet	Flour, whole grain
Oats*	Bran, flour, meal
Quinoa	Cereal, flour, whole grain
Rice (brown)	Bread, crackers, tortillas, rice cakes, whole grain
Sorghum	Flour, whole grain
Teff	Flour, whole grain
White beans*	Flour
Wild rice	Flour, whole grain, rice cakes

Note: Avoid for the first two months.

ENCOURAGEMENT FROM LESLIE

I'm now in the second month of the anti-candida diet. I feel great, and the persistent yeast infections and constant colds I've long suffered from seem to have vanished. Thus far, I've lost about sixteen pounds. Before I found you and your book, I was in the 175-pound range. I felt hopeless, depressed, and miserable. I was sick constantly, and my recurring yeast infections were not responsive to prescription medication.

I am very grateful for your book and the work you do. Your guidance has been instrumental in getting me back to health and wellness. More important, I feel great; I feel capable and competent in being my own healer, and I feel confident and empowered by my body's ability to restore itself to its optimal state.

ENCOURAGEMENT FROM ANNE

Following the recipes in the anti-candida diet showed me new ways of eating. Before the protocol, I thought cauliflower was boring, so I never ate it. After incorporating more veggies into my diet, I've learned that cauliflower is an extremely versatile vegetable and very delicious!

8

Essential Supplements

Restore Health and Vitality

Nutrition is the most important component of my anti-candida plan. Nourishing your body with foods that support your health while detoxing from foods that make you sick is the surest path to rid the body of candida.

But the body can't get everything it needs from food alone, especially if you are suffering from a severe case of candidiasis. In addition, today's agricultural practices have left soils devoid of minerals. You need to eat five to ten times what your grandparents ate to get the same nutrient value that was present in fresh produce a century ago. This is where supplementation comes in. As I have noted throughout these pages, supplements serve multiple purposes. They replace the missing vitamins and minerals in foods that have been grown in depleted soil, they support detoxification in your body, and they provide you with the nutrients, vitamins, and minerals needed for long-term health and quality aging.

While I have included specific instructions for taking the supplements I recommend, it is a good idea to work in conjunction with your health-care practitioner prior to taking any new dietary supplements. She will be able to identify any potential interactions with other supplements or prescription medications you may be taking, and identify any other risks specific to your health or medical conditions.

Before you begin taking these supplements, let's go over some basic guidelines:

- As with any specialized diet or nutrition supplementation program, you should consult your physician or health-care provider prior to starting any of the programs discussed in this book, or prior to taking any new dietary supplements. Your physician can identify any potential interactions with other supplements or prescription medications you may be taking, and any other risks that might be specific to your health or medical conditions.
- Every individual is different, and my protocol is derived from a collective assessment of thousands of clients I have seen over the years. These are suggestions, not a guarantee.
- Women who are pregnant or breast-feeding should wait until they are done breast-feeding to do my 90-day program. When in doubt, always check with your physician.
- Do not start taking an antifungal if you are not moving your bowels at least once a day. This must be corrected before you start the antifungal. See "Supplementation for Additional Needs" on page 226 for supplements you can take for constipation.
- Always purchase your supplements from reputable sources, such as a health practitioner, professional supplement companies, health food stores, or online vitamin warehouses such as vitacost .com, iherb.com, or amazon.com. In the Resources section (page 266), I list sources for all the supplements outlined in this section. The small amounts of soy in some of the products there are acceptable and are usually non-GMO. Supplements sold in drug-

stores and supermarkets often contain sugar, synthetic dyes, and fillers. Read labels to make sure they say "no added dyes, fillers, sugar, corn, or yeast."

- The abX products are my own line of supplements, which I recommend, having used them with good results for many years in clinical practice. They are a possible choice, not mandatory. What matters most is that you address the areas of imbalance that I write about in each section and use quality vitamins/supplements.
- If you live outside the United States, look for comparable products with similar ingredients to the supplements I have suggested by going online and viewing the ingredient labels of these supplements.
- Periodically check my website, annboroch.com, for the latest updates on supplement changes that pertain to this section. Some companies change their formulations, or a supplement may no longer be on the market.
- If you experience an upset stomach when taking any of the supplements that are supposed to be taken on an empty stomach, you may take them after meals. If you experience diarrhea or an allergic reaction from any supplement, stop taking it for three days, and then try taking one pill once a day to see if you tolerate it. If you do, continue to build up slowly. If you do not, discontinue the supplement permanently.
- In general, I recommend taking supplements within a half hour of finishing a meal. For those who can only swallow one or two pills at a time, take supplements right before your first bite of food instead of after the meal. This way you won't feel waterlogged. Some supplements are best taken on an empty stomach; in this case, you can take them fifteen to thirty minutes before a meal or one and a half hours after a meal.
- Remember to drink adequate amounts of water and herbal teas daily—one half of your body weight in ounces.

At first glance, you might feel overwhelmed by the need to make new food choices and take all the supplements. To ease into the program, a week before beginning, buy groceries and think about your different meal options, including what you can eat in restaurants while you're following the protocol. Order or purchase the recommended supplements for detoxifying and rebuilding your body (see Resources, page 266, for vendors). By the end of the first week, you will have started to feel better—you will be clearer, have more energy, and find that you are adjusting to the rhythm of the 90-day program.

Note: Those who have chosen to do the slow-start elimination plan will only begin the following 90-day program after eliminating all the foods listed below.

90-Day Program Overview with Supplements

FIRST MONTH: DAYS 1–30

Nutrition

- Eliminate sugars, fermented or yeast products, dairy products, refined carbohydrates, corn, gluten, trans fats, caffeine (except in white tea), and alcohol.

Antifungal (work up slowly)

Take one of the following antifungals. Choose either an herbal (preferable) or pharmaceutical antifungal based on your needs (see pages 63–65 for a more in-depth discussion):

- Candida abX, from Quintessential Healing
- Candida Cleanse, from Rainbow Light
- Candida Support, from NOW Foods
- Nystatin
- Diflucan (to jump-start only; then switch to nystatin)

As I explained in chapter 4, "Candida Detox," pharmaceutical antifungals like Diflucan and nystatin are recommended for autoimmune and cancer conditions or if you have severe anxiety and/or depression or mental illness. Diflucan can be taken to give your body a jump-start and kill off systemic fungus at the beginning of your program. After jump-starting with Diflucan, as described below, you can then switch to nystatin or an herbal antifungal.

How to Take an Herbal Antifungal

If you are taking Candida abX, Candida Cleanse, or Candida Support in pill form, start with one capsule or tablet per day after a meal and slowly increase the dosage by one capsule or tablet every three days until you reach the dose recommended on the chart on page 218. For severe cases of candida overgrowth, I suggest doubling the dose of herbal antifungals to two pills three times a day after meals for three to four months, then reduce to one pill three times a day. At this dosage you would be getting closer to the potency of nystatin.

Diflucan and nystatin are prescription drugs. You would need to find a physician who is willing to prescribe them, and take according to his directions. Below is a regimen that I have seen work for other clients, but always follow the advice of your physician.

Suggested way to take a pharmaceutical antifungal (nystatin):

For an adult, dosing of nystatin is one pill (500,000 units) taken three times a day without food half an hour before a meal. Take it with food, however, if it upsets your stomach. Work up slowly to the full dose.

Suggested way to jump-start with Diflucan, for those with cancer, autoimmune disease, or mental illness:

Ask your doctor to prescribe three 150 mg tablets. Take one pill every three days for one week.

After jump-start, switch to nystatin:

After your jump-start of three Diflucan tablets (one pill every three days), begin taking nystatin, slowly working your way up to one pill three times a day. Start off with one pill per day, and after three days, increase to one pill twice a day. After another three days, increase to one pill three times a day. Continue at this dosage for six to twelve months. For the third month, add probiotics such as 11-Strain Probiotic Powder, Flora 20-14, Ultimate Flora 30 Billion, or Garden of Life Dr. Formulated Probiotics Once Daily 30 Billion, taking them at a separate time from the nystatin.

Or you can switch to an herbal antifungal: after jump-starting with Diflucan for one week, switch to Candida abX or one of the other herbal antifungals and take as directed for a minimum of twelve months, for chronic conditions. To get the greatest benefits from the antifungal, switch to another herbal antifungal every three months. For the third month, add probiotics such as 11-Strain Probiotic Powder, Flora 20-14, or Ultimate Flora 30 Billion, taking them at a separate time from the herbal antifungal.

Notes

- If you decide to use Diflucan for more than a week, have your doctor monitor your liver enzymes.
- Antifungals can make you feel worse before you feel better. Work your dosage up slowly to allow your system to keep up with the elimination of toxins.
- If you are wheelchair-bound or bedridden, do not take pharmaceutical antifungals. Start by taking probiotics for month one, and then take Candida abX according to the instructions for herbal antifungals above.

Additional Supplements

In addition to an antifungal, I suggest the following supplements to ensure proper detoxification and repair of the body.

- **Intestinal repair formula—1 scoop in 4–6 ounces of water on an empty stomach on arising.**

These herbal and amino supplement powders contain flavonoids, phytochemicals, and antioxidants to help restore and repair the intestinal lining. It is essential to repair leaky gut, which will reduce inflammation in the body. These formulas may help with acid reflux, heartburn, ulcers, and brain fatigue, and reduce sugar and carbohydrate cravings. Take an additional scoop at bedtime if you have heartburn, gastric reflux, numerous allergies, or intense gastrointestinal symptoms.

Brands

- Repairvite and K-63, from Apex Energetics
- IntestiNEW, from ReNew Life

Vitamin C—300–700 mg of whole-food source, or 3,000 mg daily.

Buy vitamin C that contains a whole-food source or one with mineral ascorbates and/or bioflavonoids. Plain ascorbic acid crystals may irritate your stomach lining and intestines. I particularly like blends that have quercetin and bromelain to help reduce inflammation. Spread the dosage throughout the day because your body will absorb only so much at one time. Increase your dose of vitamin C slowly. If you experience diarrhea, cut back your dose. You can take powders with or without food, but it's best to take pills after a meal or snack.

Brands

- QBC Plex, from Solaray
- Aller C, from Vital Nutrients
- Dr. Schulze's Super-C Plus, tablets or powder

Blood sugar/adrenal formula—1 pill 3 times a day with food.

These herbal-vitamin supplements help balance blood sugar, assist with hypoglycemia (low blood sugar), balance highs and lows of energy throughout the day, and decrease sugar/carb cravings. They can also be used as needed after the 90-day program whenever sugar/carb cravings kick in or hypoglycemic symptoms return. If you are diabetic, during the 90-day program use an insulin-resistance formula instead, such as Glysen or Pancreas Tonic (see "Brands" below).

Brands

- Gluco abX, from Quintessential Healing
- Bio-Glycozyme Forte, from Biotics Research

High Blood Sugar and Insulin Resistance—1 capsule 3 times a day with food.

These herbal-vitamin supplements assist with high blood sugar (hyperglycemia) and insulin resistance. They can be used long-term if needed after the 90-day program. If you feel wired or anxious when taking either of these formulas, which contain glandulars, reduce dosage—skip taking your dinner dose. If symptoms continue, stop taking the product altogether and switch to a multivitamin and mineral (Life Extension Two-Per-Day Capsules, Designs for Health Complete Multi) or blood-sugar formula for prediabetes/diabetes and insulin resistance.

Brands

- Glysen, from Apex Energetics
- Pancreas Tonic, from Made in USA

Gallbladder formula—work up slowly to 1 capsule 3 times a day with food.

These herbal-vitamin supplements stimulate bile secretion, decongest the gallbladder, and help eliminate toxins from the gallbladder and liver. Use for the first month only, and then switch to a liver formula for the second and third months.

Brands

- Gallbladder abX, from Quintessential Healing
- Liv-Gall Cleanse, from Herbal Factors
- Lipo-Gen, from Metagenics

Notes

- If your gallbladder has been removed, you can still use a gallbladder formula to assist with the digestive process.
- If diarrhea or stomach upset occurs, stop taking the gallbladder formula for three days and then start up again with one pill a day, slowly working back up to three pills a day. If diarrhea occurs again, stop taking altogether and replace with a liver formula.

Vitamin E—400 IU daily.

When buying vitamin E, be sure the source is natural. Look for d-tocopherol on the label, not dl-tocopherol, which is synthetic. Also, use an E vitamin that has mixed tocopherols and tocotrienols.

Brands

- E Gems Elite, from Carlson
- familE, from Jarrow Formulas

Notes

- Do not take vitamin E if you are on blood thinners.
- If you will be having surgery, stop taking vitamin E two weeks before so your blood will clot properly.
- If you begin to bruise easily, reduce your dosage of vitamin E.

Digestive enzymes—1 after each meal (optional).

It's usually a good idea to add digestive enzymes for the first month or two of your program to make sure you're digesting, absorbing, and eliminating properly. It is especially recommended if you do not take Gluco abX or Gallbladder abX, which contain enzymes. If you have trouble digesting animal protein (burping and heartburn), buy an enzyme that contains pepsin and hydrochloric acid (HCl). If you have low blood sugar—your energy is up and down throughout the day, and you feel shaky and crabby if you skip a meal—use pancreatin, a supplement containing the pancreatic enzymes lipase, protease, and amylase. If you're a vegetarian or have mild digestive complaints, use a plant-based digestive enzyme.

Brands

- Enzy-Gest, from Priority One. A full-bodied digestive/pancreatic enzyme containing HCl, pepsin, and pancreatin.
- Digest Gold, from Enzymedica. Plant-based for vegetarians.

Ground flaxseed—1 tablespoon in 8 ounces of water.

Fiber is key to keeping your bowels moving daily, sweeping debris from the colon lining, and lowering cholesterol. Alternatively, you can put flaxseed in a smoothie, or sprinkle on salads or vegetables. Keep refrigerated after opening.

Brands

- Bob's Red Mill
- Spectrum Organic

Red clover tea—work up slowly to 4 cups daily.

This herb cleanses your bloodstream, liver, and kidneys. One heaping teaspoon of the loose herb makes one cup of tea. To make four cups of the tea, bring one quart of filtered water to a boil, and turn off the heat. Place four teaspoons of the bulk herb in a large French press, add boiling water, let the tea steep for fifteen minutes, and then slowly push the plunger down. After brewing, you can add ice cubes to make iced tea to drink throughout the day. Make sure to consume whatever amount you make the same day, or it will get moldy, even if kept in the refrigerator. You can also use organic red clover tea bags if you don't want to make a batch at a time (Celebration or Alvita are good brands).

Notes

- Do not drink red clover tea if you have grass allergies, ulcers, or acid reflux, or if you are taking blood-thinning medication. Instead, drink one cup of low-caffeine organic white tea or dandelion-root tea daily.
- Buy only organic red clover dried herb tea in bulk or tea bags. A good organic bulk supplier is Mountain Rose Herbs (see Resources, page 266).
- Some people have reported that drinking red clover tea at night keeps them awake. This is due to the cleansing effect on the bloodstream. If you experience this, it is best to finish drinking red clover tea by 5:00 p.m.

First Month: Days 1–30 Supplement Schedule

Supplement	Arising	Breakfast	Lunch	Dinner	Bedtime	After Meal*	Empty Stomach
Antifungal (dose depends on which product is used)†, ‡	X		X (½ hour before meal)	X (½ hour before meal)			X
RepairVite§	1 scoop						X
Vitamin C	Dose depends on which product is used					X (pills/ powder)	X (powder only)
Gluco abX or Glysen		1	1	1	1	X	
Gallbladder abX‡		1	1	1			X
Vitamin E (400 IU)		1				X	
Digestive enzymes (optional)		1	1	1		X	
Ground flaxseed	1 tbsp anytime during the day					X	X
Red clover tea‡	4 cups daily					X	X
Molybdenum, 150 mcg (optional)	1					X	

* After-meal supplements will digest better and make you feel less bloated if you take them right before your first bite of food rather than your last bite of food.

† Antifungal/antimicrobial: Candida abX, Candida Cleanse, pau d'arco pills, or nystatin (1 pill 3 times a day), OR pau d'arco tincture or Cleanse. Those jump-starting with Diflucan take one 150 mg tablet every 3 days for 1 week; then switch to an herbal antifungal or nystatin. Nystati can be used for up to two years for autoimmune diseases. Work up slowly to the full dose of a antifungal. If an antifungal upsets your stomach, take with a meal rather than ½ hour before meal.

‡ Start slowly with this antifungal/supplement/tea—1 pill or 1 cup for 3 days, then increase to 2 pills or 2 cups for 3 days, and so on. Do not drink red clover tea if you have grass allergies, ulcers, or acid reflux, or if you are taking blood-thinning medication.

§ RepairVite: Mix with 4–6 ounces of water. Take an additional scoop at bedtime if you have heartburn, acid reflux, numerous allergies, or intense gastrointestinal symptoms.

Molybdenum—150 mcg daily (optional).

This is a trace mineral that assists with the breakdown of acetaldehyde, a main by-product of candida. It can help alleviate die-off symptoms such as brain fog, spaciness, headaches, and vertigo. Take as needed until symptoms subside.

Brand

- Country Life

Second and Third Months: Days 31–90

Nutrition

- Eliminate sugars, fermented or yeast products, dairy products, refined carbohydrates, corn, gluten, trans fats, caffeine (except white tea), and alcohol.

Antifungal

Continue taking your antifungal at the dosage where you left off at the end of the first month. For severe cases of candida, keep the dose of Candida abX or Candida Cleanse at 2 pills 3 times a day.

Additional Supplements

Liver formula—work up slowly to 1 capsule 3 times a day with food.

These herbal formulas assist with liver detoxification by converting harmful chemicals into water-soluble substances so they can be easily eliminated in the urine and feces. Use for months two and three of your program. The liver formula replaces the Gallbladder abX or Lipo-Gen you used during the first month.

Brands

- Liver abX, from Quintessential Healing
- Daily Liver Support, from ReNew Life
- Lipo-Gen, from Metagenics

Omega-3 fish oil—1,200–1,500 mg daily with food.

Omega-3 is an essential fatty acid that is not manufactured by the body and helps decrease inflammation, feed brain and nerve cells, and support cardiovascular function. It is important to buy a brand that is free of PCBs (carcinogenic man-made chemicals used in electrical equipment and industrial processes). The brands that follow are PCB-free.

Brands

- Ultimate Omega 3 fish oil gels, from Nordic Naturals
- Elite Omega-3 Gems Fish Oil, Professional Strength, from Carlson
- OmegaGenics EPA-DHA 720, from Metagenics

Note

- Do not take fish oil if you are on blood-thinning medication. If you will be having surgery, stop taking the fish oil two weeks before so your blood will clot properly.

Blood sugar/adrenal formula—1 pill 2 times a day with food.

If you are still experiencing sugar and carbohydrate cravings and/or are hypoglycemic, stay on Gluco abX or Bio-Glycozyme Forte for days 31 to 60. However, if you feel stabilized, stop taking Gluco abX and switch to Adrenal abX (see page 222) to assist with balancing adrenal function and to give you more energy.

Brands

- OmegaGenics EPA-DHA 720, from Metagenics
- Gluco abX, from Quintessential Healing
- Bio-Glycozyme Forte, from Biotics Research

OR

Blood sugar formula for prediabetes, diabetes, or insulin resistance—1 capsule 3 times a day with food.

Keep taking Glysen or Pancreas Tonic for days 31–90 if you are diabetic or are still struggling with insulin resistance. These formulas can be used long-term if needed after the 90-day program.

Brands

- Glysen, from Apex Energetics
- Pancreas Tonic, from Made in USA

Adrenal formula—1 tablet 2 times a day with food.

These herbal vitamin supplements balance adrenal function and are useful for relieving fatigue and the effects of high stress. If you are a vegetarian, you can take Adaptocrine, Adrenal Health, or Korean red ginseng (see plant-based formulas below). If your energy levels are optimal, replace Adrenal abX with a multivitamin and mineral (Life Extension's Two-Per-Day Capsules or Designs for Health's Complete Multi).

Brand

- Adrenal abX, from Quintessential Healing

OR

Plant-based adrenal formulas, for vegetarians—1 pill 2 times a day with food.

These herbal-vitamin supplements are suitable for vegetarians. They assist with relieving fatigue and the effects of high stress and can be used long-term if needed after the 90-day program.

Brands

- Adaptocrine, from Apex Energetics
- Adrenal Health, from Gaia Herbs
- Korean red ginseng, from Prince of Peace or Imperial Elixir

Evening Primrose Oil, for women only—500 mg twice a day.

This is an omega-6 essential fatty acid that is rich in gamma linoleic acid (GLA), which assists in balancing female hormones and eliminating PMS symptoms.

Brands

- Source Naturals
- NOW Foods

Vitamin C—300–700 mg whole-food source, or 3,000 mg daily.

Buy a vitamin C that contains a whole-food source or one with mineral ascorbates and/or bioflavonoids. Plain ascorbic acid crystals will irritate the lining of your stomach and intestines. Spread out the dosage through the day because your body will absorb only so much at one time. Increase your dose of vitamin C slowly. If you experience diarrhea, cut back your dose. You can take powders with or without food, but it's best to take pills after a meal or snack.

Brands

- QBC Plex, from Solaray
- Aller C, from Vital Nutrients
- Dr. Schulze's Super-C Plus, tablets or powder

Vitamin E—400 IU daily.

When buying vitamin E, be sure the source is natural. Look for d-tocopherol on the label, not dl-tocopherol, which is synthetic. Also use an E vitamin that has mixed tocopherols and tocotrienols.

Brands

- E Gems Elite, from Carlson
- familE, from Jarrow Formulas

Notes

- Do not take vitamin E if you are on blood thinners.
- If you will be having surgery, stop taking vitamin E two weeks before so your blood will clot properly.
- If you begin to bruise easily, reduce your dosage of vitamin E.

Green food formula and/or Vegetable Alkalizer Juice.

Take an alkalizing green formula in either a pill, powder, or liquid form and/or drink Vegetable Alkalizer Juice (page 196). Even if you eat dark leafy greens each day, you need additional superfoods and greens to keep your body alkaline; to detoxify the negative effects from radiation, chemicals, and heavy metals; and to provide your body with sufficient minerals to repair itself.

Brands

- NanoGreens10, from BioPharma Scientific
- Vitamineral Green from HealthForce Nutritionals

Ground Flaxseed

Put one tablespoon of organic ground flaxseed in eight ounces of water or sprinkle on salads or vegetables. Fiber is key to keeping your bowels moving daily, sweeping debris from the colon lining, and lowering cholesterol. Keep refrigerated after opening.

Brands

- Bob's Red Mill
- Spectrum Organic

Digestive enzymes (optional)—1 after each meal.

Take for the second month only as needed (if you still have gas, bloating, heartburn, or constipation).

Red clover tea—work up slowly to 3 to 4 cups daily.

This herb cleanses your bloodstream, liver, and kidneys. One heaping teaspoon of the loose herb makes one cup of tea. To make four cups of the tea, bring one quart of filtered water to a boil, and turn off the heat. Place four teaspoons of the bulk herb in a large French press, add boiling water, let the tea steep for fifteen minutes, then slowly push the plunger down. After brewing, you can add ice cubes to make iced tea to drink throughout the day. Make sure to consume whatever amount you make the same day or it will get moldy, even if kept in the refrigerator. You can also use organic red clover tea bags if you don't want to make a batch at a time (Celebration or Alvita are good brands).

Supplement	Arising	Breakfast	Lunch	Dinner	Bedtime	After Meal*	Empty Stomach
Antifungal (dose depends on which product is used)†	X		X (½ hour before meal)	X (½ hour before meal)			X
Vitamin C	Dose depends on which product is used					X (pills/powder)	X (powder only)
Liver abX		*	*	*		X	
Vitamin E (400 IU)		*				X	
Ground flaxseed	1 tbsp anytime during the day					X	X
Red clover tea	4 cups daily					X	X
Omega 3 fish oil	*			*		X	
Evening primrose oil (women only)		*		*		X	
Adrenal abX or Adaptocrine		*	*			X	
Green food/Veg. Alkalizer Juice			X				X
Gluco abX or Glysen (optional)		*	*	*		X	
Digestive enzymes (optional)		*	*	*		X	

* After-meal supplements will digest better and make you feel less bloated if you take them right before your first bite of food rather than your last bite of food.

† Continue taking your antifungal at the dosage where you left off at the end of the first month (you may switch to a different herbal antifungal for the third month). For severe cases of candida, take 2 pills of Candida abX or Candida Cleanse 3 times a day.

Supplementation for Additional Needs

The supplements listed below are for those who have additional and/or stubborn symptoms that need to be addressed while doing the 90-day program. Add them to your daily supplementation as needed.

Elimination Problems

Constipation

Herbal laxative.

Start by taking the minimum dose on the label in the evening and see if you eliminate in the morning. If you don't, increase by one pill each night after dinner until you achieve daily elimination. The goal is to have full, normal bowel movements, not diarrhea, so adjust the dose until it is right for you. If you have taken up to four pills in the evening and are still not eliminating daily, then switch to another product. Magnesium citrate and triphala are milder formulas for constipation, and Aloe Lite and Aloe 225 are stronger.

Brands

- Magnesium citrate, from Life Extension or NOW Foods
- Aloe Lite or Aloe 225, from Bio-Design
- Triphala, from Planetary Herbals or Himalaya USA (can be used long-term)
- Naturalax #2 or #3 or Aloelax, from Nature's Way
- Dr. Christopher's Quick Colon Part 1, from Christopher's Original Formulas (use only for six months; contains addictive stimulating herbs)

Aloe vera juice.

Drink 4 ounces upon arising and 4 ounces at bedtime without food. The juice from the aloe vera plant helps reduce gastrointestinal inflammation, repair leaky gut, and alleviate constipation. The juice can be used long-term.

Brands

- Lily of the Desert
- George's Aloe Vera

Diarrhea

Psyllium seed.

This is a fiber that expands in size and helps to form normal stools.

Brand

- Herbulk, from Metagenics

Leaky Gut

In this condition, the lining of the GI tract is porous and irritated, causing food allergies, asthma, and weakened immunity. It is almost a given that most people today have mild, moderate, or severe leaky gut because of our contaminated food, air, and water supply. Those with severe cases of leaky gut, indicated by such conditions as Crohn's disease, celiac disease, diverticulitis, or ulcerative colitis, or those who are taking pain medication, may take one of the following formulas for an extended period, or as needed.

RepairVite, IntestiNEW, and Glutagenics.

These herbal-vitamin powders contain the amino acid L-glutamine, aloe vera, and deglycerized licorice. They help repair leaky gut; alleviate acid reflux, heartburn, ulcers, and brain fatigue; and help stop sugar/carb cravings.

Aloe vera juice.

Drink 4 ounces upon arising and 4 ounces at bedtime without food. The juice from the aloe vera plant helps reduce gastrointestinal inflammation, repair leaky gut, and alleviate constipation. The juice can be used long-term.

Brands

- Lily of the Desert
- George's Aloe Vera

Endefen and Intestinal Repair Complex.

These powdered herbal-vitamin formulas support the healing of an inflamed gastric lining and promote the growth of beneficial bacteria. They are good remedies for Crohn's disease, irritable bowel syndrome, and ulcerative colitis.

Thyroid Support

The largest endocrine gland in the body, the thyroid sits in the neck. It is primarily responsible for regulating metabolism. Signs of an underactive thyroid (hypothyroidism) include depression, weight gain, hair loss, puffy eyes and face, constipation, skin problems, headaches, poor circulation, fatigue, and loss of the outer third of the eyebrows. In contrast, hyperthyroidism is an autoimmune condition in which the thyroid produces too much of the hormone thyroxine. The most common form is Graves' disease, which can progress into hypothyroidism. Before addressing a thyroid imbalance, it is critical to address weak adrenal function and candida overgrowth as I have described throughout the book.

Eating seaweed (see Resources, page 266) is the best first step to balancing your thyroid and can be started at the outset of your 90-day program. Seaweed is an excellent food source of iodine as well as minerals that can help optimize thyroid function and offset the negative effects of radiation and heavy metals. Iodine is needed by the thyroid to make thyroxine. If it cannot be produced, thyroid function will be decreased, resulting in hypothyroidism. The typical Western diet is now deficient in iodine because of depleted soils, poor diets, and a decrease in the use of table salt amid sodium concerns.

If thyroid balance is not achieved, consider replacing seaweed with (or adding) Thyroid abX or GTA supplements, or asking your doctor for a prescription for Armour or Nature-Throid. When using any thyroid supplements or medication, make sure to have a blood test done every three to six months to monitor your thyroid markers.

Those with Graves' disease and Hashimoto's disease might want to avoid iodine. Check with your doctor or health practitioner.

Thyroid formulas.

These herbal-vitamin supplements are designed to balance thyroid function and are particularly beneficial for those with autoimmune thyroid conditions, such as Hashimoto's disease. These formulas can be used long-term if needed.

Brands

- Thyroid abX, from Quintessential Healing
- GTA or GTA Forte, from Biotics Research

Notes

- Do not take any thyroid supplements if you are currently taking pharmaceutical thyroid medication.
- If you notice signs of hyperthyroidism—sudden weight loss, insomnia, restlessness, rapid heartbeat, sweating, increased appetite, goiter—while taking one of these supplements, stop taking it or reduce the dosage. Have your doctor check your thyroid markers by doing blood work.

Weight-Gain Remedies

If you are having trouble keeping weight on, here are some suggestions. With each meal, eat a small amount of gluten-free grains (specifically brown rice) from the "Foods to Eat" list. Eat more winter squashes, such as pumpkin, butternut, and acorn, and eat avocado, organic pasture-raised butter or ghee, nuts, and nut butters daily (small amounts at one time). Make a protein smoothie with the protein powder listed below, using unsweetened almond, coconut, or hemp milk. Add one tablespoon of melted raw coconut oil, one tablespoon of almond or macadamia nut butter, and a banana (allowed during the first three months for those who need to gain weight).

Whey powders.

These high-grade whey powders are made from grass-fed, hormone-free cows. One formula has colostrum for extra immune support. These products are allowed for the purpose of weight gain. Those sensitive to dairy might not tolerate them well.

Brands

- NanoProPRP Immune, from BioPharma Scientific
- The True Whey, from Source Naturals

ENCOURAGEMENT FROM TOM

When I first gave up alcohol, I struggled to control my eating. My body was already taken over by candida, and I had ALL of the symptoms in your book. After your three-month detox, I can say I have eliminated 90 percent of my symptoms. Continuing on your food program, I've also lost a total of 30 pounds!

PART III

A Lifelong Cure

9

The Maintenance Plan

Keeping Your Mycobiome in Balance

After completing the 90-day plan of nutrition and supplementation, you should feel great. Now that your body is in a balanced state, it's important to maintain your new healthy habits; candida overgrowth can come back even more virulently if you begin eating junk food or overindulging in occasional "cheat" foods. Continue to avoid foods that contain sugar, dairy, yeast, corn, gluten, soy, and refined carbohydrates, and avoid drinking alcohol. You can keep your diet clean by eating the foods on the "Foods to Eat to Maintain Health" list at least 80 percent of the time and eating the foods on the "Foods to Eat Infrequently or Not at All" list only 20 percent of the time or less. One way to achieve this is to stick to the lists and eat healthily from Mondays through Fridays, and let yourself eat a little bit less rigidly on the weekends.

If you have a chronic condition, such as an autoimmune disease or cancer, it's important to continue taking a small dose of an herbal antifungal compound every day; it takes longer than 90 days to eradicate yeast overgrowth from the system. It's also a good idea to take digestive enzymes during stressful periods such as times of travel and during holidays, or when eating poorly or going to bed on a full stomach.

For those of you who are not challenged with these conditions but feel that unhealthy lifestyle habits and high stress might creep back in, it's a good idea to take ongoing maintenance doses of Candida abX (one pill two times a day), Candida Cleanse (one pill two times a day), and Candida Support (one pill two times a day). Rotate these products every three months to make sure you don't become immune to any one of them. For those who are able to maintain a healthy diet, I suggest replacing your antifungal with a probiotic and taking that every day to keep your digestive system and yeast levels in balance. Specifics about probiotics are discussed later in this chapter.

Continue to drink red clover tea or white tea each week, as it clears environmental toxins and removes stress hormones from the bloodstream. Stop drinking red clover tea for a month three times a year so that you don't become allergic to it, or switch to white or dandelion root tea during that month. You can reduce your intake of red clover tea to one to two cups three or four times a week, and drink three to four cups when you are under stress and/or your diet is poor.

Finally, now that you have completed the 90-day cycle, you will be adding foods back into your diet that you haven't eaten in a while. If you notice intolerances and reactions after eating these foods, such as a rapid pulse (90 to 180 beats per minute), fatigue, itching internally or externally, hives, gas, bloating, headaches, or other symptoms, eliminate those foods. This is a clear sign your body does not want you to eat them!

FOODS TO EAT TO MAINTAIN HEALTH

(Eat at Least 80 Percent of the Time)

Animal protein—antibiotic- and hormone-free, as much as possible

Beef, buffalo, lamb, and venison (grass-fed; eat once a week with greens, not with starchy vegetables, beans, or grains)

Chicken, duck, and turkey

Eggs (organic or pasture-raised, if possible)

Fish (limit shellfish to once or twice a month)

Grains—whole and unrefined only

Amaranth

Breads (gluten-, sugar-, dairy-, and yeast-free)

Brown, black, or wild rice (limit to 2–3 times a week)

Buckwheat

Crackers (brown rice and flax; limit to 2–3 times a week)

Millet

Oats (gluten-free)

Pasta (gluten- and corn-free; limit to once a week)

Quinoa

Sorghum

Tapioca

Teff

Yucca

Oils—cold-pressed only

Almond oil (can be used for cooking)

Avocado oil (can be used for cooking)

Coconut oil (can be used for cooking)

Flaxseed oil (not for cooking)

Grapeseed oil (can be used for cooking)

Hempseed oil (not for cooking)

Olive oil (can be used for cooking)

Pistachio oil (not for cooking)

Red palm fruit oil (can be used for cooking, low heat only)

Safflower oil (can be used for cooking)

Sesame oil (can be used for cooking)

Sunflower-seed oil (can be used for cooking)

Walnut oil (not for cooking)

Note: At restaurants, eat what is served; be more careful when using oils at home.

Nuts and seeds—raw/unroasted if commercial; may toast your own

Almonds
Brazil
Cashews
Chestnuts
Chia seeds
Flaxseeds
Hazelnuts
Hempseeds
Macadamia
Nut butters (all except peanut butter; nut butters can be dry-roasted)
Pecans
Pine nuts
Pistachios
Pumpkin seeds and pumpkin-seed butter
Sesame seeds (also raw tahini butter)
Sunflower seeds and sunflower-seed butter
Walnuts

Note: Limit quantity to a small handful at a time, and chew thoroughly.

Dairy—antibiotic- and hormone-free only

Butter (small amounts, unsalted; preferably organic from grass-fed cows)
Clarified butter (ghee, organic)
Goat and sheep cheeses (raw, once or twice a month)

Note: Pregnant and nursing women should not eat raw dairy products.

Vegetables—should make up 60 percent of your daily diet; dark-green leafy vegetables and cruciferous vegetables are most important

All except mushrooms, potatoes, and corn.

Condiments

Apple cider vinegar (raw, unfiltered only—store in refrigerator)
Bragg Liquid Aminos (unfermented soy sauce; only acceptable soy product)
Dill relish (Bubbies, made without vinegar)
Dry mustard (or small amounts of mustard made with apple cider vinegar)
Fresh herbs (basil, parsley, etc.)
Mayonnaise (small amounts made with safflower oil) or use Healthy Mayonnaise (recipe on page 179)

Original Coconut Aminos, Coconut Secret

Pepper

Rice vinegar (unseasoned and unsweetened only—store in the refrigerator)

Sea salt

Spices (without sugar, MSG, or additives; favor ginger and turmeric, which are anti-inflammatory)

Beverages

Bragg apple cider vinegar drinks (Ginger Spice, Limeade, and Sweet Stevia only)

Fresh coconut water (only during or right after exercise; there are 14 grams of sugar in a can)

Green tea, caffeinated or decaffeinated

Herbal teas (red clover, peppermint, etc.)

Suja Lemon Love lemon juice drink

Unsweetened almond, coconut, or hemp milk

Unsweetened mineral water (Gerolsteiner, Perrier)

Water—filtered, purified, or distilled only

Beans and Legumes

All except soybeans, tofu, or tempeh (organic, small amounts)

Miscellaneous:

Cacao powder (raw, unsweetened)

Carob (unsweetened)

Cocoa powder (unsweetened)

Coconut butter (organic)

Coconut yogurt (unsweetened)

Dill pickles (Bubbies, made without vinegar)

Gums/mints (sweetened with lo han, stevia, or xylitol)

Homemade fermented foods

Salsa (without sugar or vinegar, except apple cider vinegar)

Sauerkraut (Bubbies, made without vinegar)

Fruits (1–2 fruits a day):

All berries

All citrus fruits

All dried fruits (apricots, dates, figs, raisins, cranberries, prunes; limit to 1–2 times per month, as they are high in sugar)

All melons

Apples

Apricots

Avocado*

Bananas

Cherries

Coconut (small amounts of coconut water, as it is high in sugar)

Grapes (small amounts, as they are high in sugar)

Kiwis

Lemons, limes*

Mangoes

Nectarines

Papayas

Peaches

Pears

Persimmon

Pineapples

Plums

Pomegranates

* Avocado and lemon or lime juice can be in addition to your 1–2 fruits per day.

Sweeteners

Chicory root (Just Like Sugar)

Lo han kuo (monk fruit extract)

Stevia

Xylitol (small amounts; Ultimate Sweetener, Xyla)

FOODS TO EAT INFREQUENTLY OR NOT AT ALL

(Eat 20 Percent of the Time or Less)

Animal Protein

Bacon (except gluten-free turkey bacon without nitrates and hormones)

Hot dogs (except gluten-free chicken or turkey hot dogs without nitrates or hormones; small amounts because they are high in sodium)

Processed and packaged meats

Sausages (except gluten-free chicken and turkey without added sugar, hormones, and nitrates)

Shellfish, farmed fish, GMO salmon, tuna (all: toro, albacore, ahi, etc., including canned)

Oils

- Canola oil (small amounts okay)
- Corn oil
- Cottonseed oil
- Partially hydrogenated or hydrogenated oils
- Peanut oil
- Soy oil

Vegetables

- Corn
- Potatoes

Nuts and Seeds

- Peanuts, peanut butter

Dairy

- Buttermilk
- Cheeses (all, including cottage and cream cheese)
- Cow's milk
- Goat's milk
- Ice cream
- Margarine
- Sour cream
- Yogurt (unless plain in raw goat dairy or coconut base, antibiotic- and hormone-free)

Grains

- Barley
- Breads (refined)
- Cereals (dry, except gluten- and sugar-free)
- Corn
- Crackers (white flour, gluten)
- Farro
- Kamut
- Pasta (except corn- and gluten-free)
- Pastries
- Popcorn
- Rye
- Spelt
- Triticale
- Wheat (refined and whole)
- White flours
- White rice

Condiments

Gravy

Jams and jellies

Ketchup

Mayonnaise (except small amounts with safflower oil) or Healthy Mayonnaise (recipe on page 179)

Pickles

Relish

Salad dressing, unless sugar-free and made with apple cider vinegar or unsweetened rice vinegar

Sauces with vinegars and sugar

Soy sauce, ponzu, and tamari sauce

Spices that contain yeast, sugar, or additives, such as MSG

Beans and Legumes

Soybeans (tofu, tempeh)

Miscellaneous

Candy

Chocolate (dark, if you do indulge)

Cookies

Doughnuts

Fast food and fried foods

Fruit strips

Gelatin

Gum (unless sweetened with lo han, stevia, or xylitol)

Jerky (beef, turkey)

Lozenges/mints (unless sweetened with lo han, stevia, or xylitol)

Muffins

Pastries

Pizza

Popcorn

Processed food (TV dinners, etc.)

Smoked, dried, pickled, and cured foods

Beverages

Alcohol

Coffee, including decaffeinated (if you do indulge, drink espresso, organic only, 1 cup per day maximum)

Energy drinks (Red Bull, Gatorade, etc.)

Fruit juices

Kefir (pasteurized)

Kombucha

Rice milk

Sodas (diet and regular)

Soy milk

Fruits

All dried fruits (apricots, dates, figs, raisins, sweetened cranberries, prunes, etc.)

All juices (sweetened or unsweetened)

Sweeteners

Agave nectar/syrup (Nectevia)

Artificial sweeteners, such as aspartame (Nutrasweet), acesulfame potassium, saccharin, and sucralose (Splenda)

Barley malt

Brown rice syrup

Brown sugar

Coconut nectar/sugar

Corn syrup, dextrose, maltodextrin

Erythritol (Nectresse, Swerve, Truvia)

Fructose, and products sweetened with fruit juice

Honey (raw and processed)

Maltitol

Mannitol

Maple syrup

Molasses

Raw or evaporated cane juice crystals

Sorbitol

White sugar

Yacon syrup

What if I Need to Take an Antibiotic?

There are those critical times when you may need to take an antibiotic for a bacterial infection such as pneumonia, staph, strep, or *H. pylori*. If your doctor prescribes an antibiotic and you choose to take it, ask for Diflucan (fluconazole), one tablet, to take after you finish the antibiotic. Take probiotics such as Flora 20-14, 11-Strain Probiotic Powder, or Ultimate Flora 50 Billion while on the antibiotic, but at a different time of the day. After your antibiotic course, take one Diflucan tablet. Take the probiotics while you're taking the Diflucan, but at a different time, and continue the probiotics for one more month. Then switch to two months of herbal antifungals such as Candida abX or Candida Cleanse.

Doctors usually don't offer antifungals, but your physician might be willing to prescribe one if you ask. If you can't get Diflucan, take one month of probiotics while on the antibiotics and then switch to taking the antifungal you have been taking while on the program (e.g., Candida abX, Candida Cleanse, or Candida Support).

If you are not ambulatory, but have started the antifungal and supplement protocol and are feeling stronger and eliminating daily, you should be able to handle Diflucan. However, if you are weak or haven't started the program yet, use only the probiotics.

Supplementation for Quality Aging

To keep yourself balanced and to experience quality aging, follow the recommendations below after you finish your 90-day program.

Fourth Month and Ongoing

(See table, page 249)

Nutrition

- Eat foods from the "Foods to Eat to Maintain Health" list (page 235). Slowly introduce any new foods back into your diet. If you have a poor reaction, stay away from that food or indulge in it less frequently.
- Avoid the foods on the "Foods to Eat Infrequently or Not at All" list (page 238) or eat them only 20 percent of the time or less.

Supplements

Probiotics—dairy-free strains of acidophilus and bifidus.

Probiotics replace and balance bacteria in the GI tract. Take as directed on the bottle, typically twice a day on an empty stomach. If you are disciplined by nature and can maintain a healthy diet and minimal stress, taking the probiotic for the rest of your life should be sufficient to keep you free from candida overgrowth. However, for most people, stress and poor diet more often prevail. In these cases, to stay balanced it is best to take a probiotic as well as an herbal antifungal for the rest of your life, as described below.

Brands

- Flora 20-14, from Innate Response (refrigerate)
- 11-Strain Probiotic Powder, from Custom Probiotics (refrigerate)
- Ultimate Flora Extra Care 30 Billion Go Pack, from ReNew Life
- Dr. Ohhira's Probiotics Original Formula, from Essential Formulas
- Dr. Formulated Probiotics Once Daily 30 Billion, from Garden of Life

Herbal antifungal—only for those who have continual high stress and do not maintain a clean diet.

As stated above, taking a probiotic for the rest your life (without an antifungal) is sufficient if you can maintain a clean diet and low stress levels. Those who find it too challenging to do this would do best to take a probiotic as well as an antifungal to stay balanced. To make sure that you don't become immune to an antifungal formula, remember to rotate formulas (Candida abX, Candida Support, and Candida Cleanse) every three months, as described on page 234. Take the antifungal for three months, and then take probiotics for a month. Continue this cycle for life. Alternatively, you can take both antifungals and probiotics in the same month, but at different times of the day. Take your antifungal with meals, and take your probiotic either before sleep or between meals on an empty stomach.

Multivitamin-mineral supplement.

A good multivitamin-mineral supplement will compensate for some of the nutrients that are missing in your diet. Make sure your source has chelated minerals (minerals bound with amino acids to improve digestion) and no iron. If you are anemic and need additional iron, use food-based brands; synthetic iron can be toxic to the brain. Hemagenics (made by Metagenics) and Thorne Research's iron bisglycinate, which are both nonconstipating, are good sources.

Brands

- Two-Per-Day Capsules, from Life Extension
- DFH Complete Multi, from Designs for Health

B-complex vitamins (optional).

If you are taking a one-a-day multivitamin-mineral supplement as opposed to a brand that you are supposed to take twice or three times a day, you will need to take an extra B-complex supplement. B-complex vitamins are a must for vegetarians because certain B vitamins are lacking in a vegetarian diet.

Brands

- B Complex Plus, from Pure Encapsulations
- Glucogenics, from Metagenics
- B-, from Jarrow Formulas

Vitamin C—300–700 mg whole-food source or 2,000 mg daily.

Buy a vitamin C that contains a whole-food source or one with mineral ascorbates and/or bioflavonoids. Plain ascorbic acid crystals will irritate the lining of your stomach and intestines. Spread out the dosage through the day because your body will absorb only so much at one time. Increase your dose of vitamin C slowly. If you experience diarrhea, cut back your dose. You can take powders with or without food, but it's best to take pills after a meal or snack. A multivitamin-mineral supplement does contain vitamin C, but not enough for quality aging.

Brands

- QBC Plex, from Solaray
- Aller C, from Vital Nutrients
- Dr. Schulze's Super-C Plus, tablets or powder

Vitamin E—400 IU daily.

When buying vitamin E, be sure the source is natural. Look for d-tocopherol on the label, not dl-tocopherol, which is synthetic. Also, use an E vitamin that has mixed tocopherols and tocotrienols. A multivitamin-mineral supplement does contain vitamin E, but not enough for quality aging.

Brands

- E Gems Elite, from Carlson
- familE, from Jarrow Formulas

Notes

- Do not take vitamin E if you are on blood thinners.
- If you will be having surgery, stop taking vitamin E two weeks prior so your blood will clot properly.
- If you begin to bruise easily, reduce your dosage of vitamin E.

Green food formula and/or Vegetable Alkalizer Juice.

Take an alkalizing green formula in either a pill, powder, or liquid form and/or drink Vegetable Alkalizer Juice (see page 196). Even if you eat dark leafy greens each day, you need additional superfoods and greens to keep your body alkaline; to detoxify the negative effects from radiation, chemicals, and heavy metals; and to provide your body with sufficient minerals to repair itself.

Brands

- NanoGreens10, from BioPharma Scientific
- Vitamineral Green, from HealthForce Nutritionals

Free-form amino acid complex—2 pills upon arising; if it irritates your stomach, take after breakfast.

Amino acids are the building blocks of protein, responsible for repairing and regenerating every cell, tissue, and organ in your body. They also assist the liver's detoxification process and are the precursors to neurotransmitters such as serotonin, dopamine, and epinephrine.

Brands

- AminoBlend 740 mg, from Douglas Labs
- Max-Amino Caps, from Country Life
- Free Aminos, from Nutricology

Omega-3 fish oil—1,200–1,500 mg daily with food.

This essential fatty acid is not manufactured by the body. It helps decrease inflammation, feed brain and nerve cells, and support cardiovascular function. It is important to buy a brand that is free of PCBs (carcinogenic man-made chemicals used in electrical equipment and industrial processes). The brands I have listed below are PCB-free.

Brands

- OmegaGenics EPA-DHA 720, from Metagenics
- Ultimate Omega-3 fish oil gels, from Nordic Naturals
- Elite Omega-3 Gems Fish Oil, Professional Strength, from Carlson

Note

- Do not take fish oil if you are on blood-thinning medication. If you will be having surgery, stop taking the fish oil two weeks before so your blood will clot properly.

Evening primrose oil, for women only—500 mg twice a day.

This omega-6 essential fatty acid source is rich in gamma linoleic acid (GLA), which assists in balancing female hormones and eliminating PMS symptoms.

Brands

- Jarrow Formulas
- NOW Foods

Vitamin D3—1,000 IU.

Vitamin D is a fat-soluble vitamin that has many functions, from contributing to bone health to supporting immune function. Even though the body manufactures vitamin D when skin is exposed to ultraviolet radiation from the sun, most people today are found to have low levels. Vitamin D3 (cholecalciferol) is the best supplement form to take. You can easily have your blood tested to see if your vitamin D levels are out of range and how much you need. Those with autoimmune diseases should take higher amounts—4,000–8,000 IU daily—to ensure that their blood levels are in the range of 60–80 ng/mL. Those taking higher amounts of vitamin D3 may want to combine it with vitamin K2. Make sure to test blood levels every three to six months if you take doses of vitamin D3 higher than 2,000 IU daily.

Brands

- Vitamin D3, from Jarrow
- Vitamin D3, from Life Extension
- D-Mulsion liquid drops, from Biotics Research

Ground flaxseed.

Put one tablespoon of organic ground flaxseed in eight ounces of water or sprinkle on salads or vegetables. Fiber is key in keeping your bowels moving daily, sweeping debris from the colon lining, and lowering cholesterol. Keep refrigerated after opening.

Brand

- Bob's Red Mill
- Spectrum Organic

Recapturing Your Vitality

You now have everything you need to begin your journey of redefining your lifestyle habits so that you can feel vibrantly healthy again. This program will help you to look and feel your best and give you the energy and motivation necessary to fulfill your goals and dreams. Just remember that your body cannot take care of itself. You need to keep up the required maintenance, just as you regularly change the oil in your car to keep it running smoothly.

The secret is to keep your mindset away from deprivation and focus on the primary purpose of this program—to remove infection and inflammation from your body so you can recapture your energy, clarity, and vitality. Ninety days is a very short period of time in which to do this. As you progress, you will enjoy hearing the comments from your family, friends, and colleagues about how great you look. Though this may be gratifying, the best part is that you will feel great inside too!

Fourth Month and Ongoing Supplement Schedule

Supplement	Arising	Breakfast	Lunch	Dinner	Bedtime	After Meal*	Empty Stomach
Probiotics or Antifungal†	X				X		X
Vitamin C	Dose depends on which product is used					X (pills/ powder)	X (powder only)
Multivitamin-mineral	Dose depends on which product is used						X
Amino acid complex	†						X
Vitamin E (400 IU)		*					X
Vitamin D3 (2,000 IU)		X				X	
Green food/ Veg. Alkalizer Juice			X				X
Ground flaxseed meal	1 tbsp anytime during the day					X	X
Omega-3 fish oil		*		*		X	
Evening primrose oil (women only)		*		*		X	
Red clover tea‡	2–4 cups, 3 or 4 times a week					X	X
Digestive enzyme (optional)		*	*	*		X	
B-complex (optional)		*				X	

* After-meal supplements will digest better and make you feel less bloated if you take them right before your first bite of food versus your last bite of food.

† Probiotics: 11-Strain Probiotic Powder, Flora 20-14, Ultimate Flora RTS 15 billion, or Primal Defense Ultra (amount indicated on bottle when arising and at bedtime). If you will be alternating probiotics with antifungals on different months, when using the antifungal, take one pill three times a day half an hour before a meal, or after meals if it upsets your stomach. Check probiotics label to see if refrigeration is required.

‡ Continue to drink red clover tea each week, but stop drinking it for a month three times a year so you don't become allergic to it, or switch to dandelion root tea during that month.

ENCOURAGEMENT FROM TERESA

I'm a singer, fifty-seven years old. In my thirties, I started having issues with upper respiratory, sinus, and digestive problems. It wasn't debilitating, but annoying. My voice kept getting worse and worse until it was even difficult to talk without effort. When I tried to sing I could not go up the scale and would have involuntary pitch changes that sounded terrible. I went through vocal cord surgery and vocal injections. I started the anti-candida diet and have been taking Candex. Now, just eight months later, I can sing again; and I sound great! I cannot believe that this was the problem all along.

10

Day 91 and Beyond

You've learned that once you take charge of your health, you can bring candida back into balance within 90 days or less. You'll be amazed at how much better you feel; how you won't miss the nagging aches and ailments. It's time to celebrate the end of your symptoms. *Staying* in balance, however, takes vigilance. You don't want to revert to old habits and find symptoms and ailments returning. Continue to build on the healthy lifestyle you have created.

FAQs

On day 91 of your anti-candida program, you'll still have questions. The following FAQs are based on those I receive regularly from my clients.

Q: I've read different opinions about the health value of coffee. Why do you advise avoiding it on your program?

A: I prefer that everyone avoid coffee on the 90-day anti-candida program to give the adrenal glands a rest and to discover your baseline energy level.

Caffeine elevates adrenal hormones, which then elevate blood sugar, which then feeds candida. Coffee is also one of the most chemically treated food products in the world, and decaffeinated coffee is even worse. A mold-free brand such as Bulletproof would be a better choice if you drink it. During your 90-day program I do allow organic white tea and unfermented green tea, which contain low levels of caffeine that won't disrupt the endocrine system and are an excellent blood cleanser. After your program it's fine to consume one or two cups of organic coffee. Drinking higher amounts will put added stress on your adrenal glands.

Q: Can I drink kombucha after 90 days?

A: No. Kombucha (fermented, sweetened black or green tea) contains nonbeneficial bacteria and yeasts, which will aggravate candida. It also contains small amounts of alcohol.

Q: Is any amount of soy acceptable?

A: Supplements with lecithin and phosphatidylcholine derived from soy are acceptable, and Bragg Liquid Aminos are fine. Avoid all other soy products for 90 days, including soy isolates found in protein powders and bars. For those sensitive to soy, substitute Coconut Aminos for Bragg Liquid Aminos. Ninety percent of soy in the United States is genetically modified.

Q: Is it safe to eat fish?

A: Cautiously, I say yes. I do not recommend eating king mackerel, swordfish, tilefish, shark, or tuna of any kind (albacore, ahi/yellowfin, toro/bluefin) because they contain high levels of mercury. Radiation from the Fukushima power plant has also contaminated some of the fish supply. When eating fish, look for wild-caught—many farmed fisheries use antibiotics and pesticides—and nothing genetically modified. Download the app Seafood Watch or visit the site Cleanfish.com to see what kinds of fish are sustainable in your area and which brands to purchase.

Q: I read online that eating leftovers is bad for candida, because food can get moldy, even if just sitting overnight. Is this a cause for concern?

A: I feel eating leftovers from the night before is acceptable. Food more than one or two days old will get moldy and aggravate candida. Frozen foods are more complicated. For example, fresh poultry can last for 9 months to a year in the freezer, hamburger 3–4 months, and cooked leftovers 2–6 months. For complete guidelines go to foodsafety.gov, a website established by the US Department of Health and Human Services.

Q: Can I eat gluten-free grains and pseudo-grains (amaranth, buckwheat, millet, quinoa, teff, wild rice) on an anti-candida diet?

A: Yes. I like to incorporate as many foods as possible to give variety, and I feel there are benefits to most food groups. To keep carbohydrates low, stick to one or two portions a day; otherwise yeast will continue to be fed. Limit brown rice and brown rice food products to two to three times a week because of its high carbohydrate content, which will continue to elevate blood sugar and feed candida.

To make grains more digestible, rinse and soak grains for thirty minutes to one hour prior to cooking. However, if, like many, you are challenged with a hectic schedule, soaking is not a must, but at least rinse the grains to remove any dirt or mold.

Some people with chronic inflammatory conditions such as those with an autoimmune disease might feel better staying off grains for one to three months.

Q: Why is corn not acceptable?

A: Corn is not included on the anti-candida diet because it converts rapidly into sugar, which will feed yeast. Also, the majority of corn is genetically modified.

Q: What can I do if I'm losing too much weight on your program?

A: If you are losing too much weight, add avocado, organic grass-fed unsalted butter, raw nuts and nut butters, coconut oil, winter squashes, and protein shakes using egg white, hemp, or brown rice protein powder, and eat a gluten-free grain at each meal. To slow down your metabolism, eat three meals a day and avoid snacking. If you are still losing weight, consider a high-grade whey protein powder such as True Whey by Source Naturals. Keep in mind that whey is dairy, which can cause gastrointestinal distress for some people.

Q: Can I eat products with nutritional yeast?

A: No. Even though there are B vitamins and minerals in nutritional yeast, it can create an allergy response and aggravate candida.

Q: Can I have tamari sauce?

A: No. Even if they're gluten-free, I like to keep soy products to a minimum, since 90 percent of soy is genetically modified. Bragg

Liquid Aminos is the only soy product that is acceptable on the program.

Q: I've heard about the benefits of resistant starch. What is it, and do I need to eat raw potatoes and green (unripe) bananas?

A: Resistant starch is a carbohydrate that is not digested in the small intestine and enters the colon, where it ferments, feeds beneficial bacteria, and helps to create a short-chain fatty acid called butyrate, which improves insulin sensitivity metabolism, and reduces inflammation. But no, I don't feel you need to eat raw potatoes and green bananas. You will get the benefits of resistant starch from eating beans, grains, and vegetables.

Q: What are prebiotics, and how are they different from probiotics?

A: Prebiotics are indigestible dietary fibers that are food or fertilizer for probiotics (good bacteria) to flourish and grow. You can increase your prebiotic intake by eating artichokes, onions, leeks, garlic, cabbage, sweet potato, asparagus, chicory root, and green apples.

Q: What is the difference between the Paleo, GAP, FODMAP, and gluten-free diets and the anti-candida diet?

A: There are many diet programs that advocate avoiding certain foods to promote wellness. The main difference with an anti-candida diet is that it removes foods that feed infection (candida, parasites, viruses, bacteria), thus reducing inflammation.

Q: I love carbs and sweets. Can I do your program?

A: Yes, you can do the program. It will be easier than you think; as candida overgrowth and blood sugar imbalances are addressed, cravings disappear. Candida abX, an herbal antifungal, and Gluco abX, a blood sugar formula, will help your body and brain become more balanced. You will not have to rely solely upon willpower.

Q: How do I stay tenacious and not give in to emotional eating?

A: A major benefit of the program is that after the first week or two, your chemistry is more balanced, which will improve emotional stability. Remind yourself that food is about obtaining fuel to run the body. Food is not about pacifying unhealthy emotions. The Emotional Freedom Technique (EFT), also known as tapping, can help with emotional eating. Go to YouTube and type in "EFT Julie Schiffman." She has many free videos to help with emotions that are keeping you unhappy. Realize you are making a choice to eat healthy. This program is short-lived, so make it a "want to" versus a "have to." You will be so proud of yourself after 90 days!

Q: Can I do this program if I'm vegan?

A: Eating a vegan diet does make it challenging to adhere to the 90-day protocol. Protein helps balance blood sugar levels, and if your only protein sources are beans/legumes and grains—both of which are high in carbohydrates—you will continue to feed candida. My best advice is to make sure you balance out starchy vegetables with plenty of leafy and cruciferous vegetables, and stay away from unnecessary carbohydrates as much as possible.

Supplements, Antifungals, Medications

Q: Do I need to get a prescription for Diflucan (fluconazole) or nystatin to do your program?

A: No. You do not need Diflucan or nystatin tablets to do my program. Herbal antimicrobials such as Candida abX are my preferred choice, so you can easily get started on your program. They also have some advantages over prescription antifungals because they address parasites and bacteria as well, which are common in those suffering with leaky gut and dysbiosis. I recommend Diflucan and nystatin, if you can obtain them from a physician, for those who have autoimmune diseases, chronic conditions, or severe candidiasis. Diflucan is ten times more potent than an herbal antifungal, and one pill every other day, with a total of three pills, can jump-start removing systemic candida overgrowth. Nystatin is five times more potent than an herbal antifungal and targets the gastrointestinal tract. I do not prescribe pharmaceuticals.

Q: What course of action is best if I have to take a course of antibiotics?

A: If you take antibiotics, be sure to add in probiotics (15 to 30 billion per capsule twice daily). Take probiotics on an empty stomach at a different time from when you take your antibiotics, which are best taken with food. See if your physician will prescribe one Diflucan pill (100 or 150 mg) to offset the antibiotics' destruction of beneficial bacteria. Take Diflucan the day after finishing your antibiotics. Then wait one more day and take two months of herbal antifungals such as Candida abX or Candida Cleanse. If you can't obtain Diflucan, start taking the herbal antifungals the day after your last antibiotic. You can continue with probiotics, but it is not necessary. The most important factor is to take an herbal antifungal to make sure candida overgrowth does not come back more virulently.

Q: If I'm taking medication, can I still do your program?

A: Yes. Make sure to check with your doctor first about any possible drug-supplement interactions. Those on blood-thinning medication such as Coumadin (warfarin) will need to be monitored because supplements such as vitamin E and fish oil will thin the blood.

Q: I've heard from various health sources that I should take vitamin K along with vitamin D to allow the vitamin D to be absorbed. Do you feel vitamin K is necessary?

A: Taking vitamin K along with vitamin D is optional. If you take higher amounts—3,000 to 5,000 IU or more—vitamin K2 (under 100 mcg) is advisable to allow better absorption and ensure that calcium is distributed properly, to bone rather than arteries. Some multivitamins and minerals contain vitamin K, so additional amounts are not needed if taking these.

Q: Why is staying on herbal antifungals and probiotics important after finishing your program?

A: Because there are times when you will eat inflammatory foods such as gluten, dairy, or sugar, or drink alcohol. In addition, we are all exposed to heavy metals in our food, air, and water, which wipe out beneficial bacteria in the gastrointestinal tract. Protecting your entire microbiome (including your mycobiome) for the rest of your life is great preventive medicine. To age with quality,

I recommend rotating every three to four months between herbal antimicrobials such as Candida abX, Candida Cleanse, or comparable products. You can reduce your dose to one or two pills a day. During times of travel, stress, or when your diet veers off, increase to three pills a day. If you maintain a 95 percent or better healthy diet, lifetime probiotics are sufficient. I would suggest alternating between two brands every three to four months.

Q: Is it okay to have food-based supplements containing *Saccharomyces cerevisiae* (a common source of B vitamins)?

A: I prefer no food-based supplements that contain yeast during the 90-day program; it can create an allergy response and slow down your progress.

Q: What can I do if I experience leg cramps?

A: If you experience leg cramps, add a mineral supplement. Many people have low magnesium levels, and supplementation will alleviate cramps. Take one or two magnesium glycinate pills at bedtime, or use a magnesium citrate powder like Natural Vitality's Raspberry Lemon Calm, which will also benefit those who are constipated. Start with the smallest dose recommended so you don't experience diarrhea. Designs for Health's Complete Mineral Complex is another option for leg cramps.

Detoxification

Q: How do I know if I'm allergic to red clover tea or a supplement?

A: If you feel itchy externally and internally, and/or you swell up with hives that persist after more than a few days, than you are having an allergic response. Stop that supplement or tea for three days and let your body normalize. Try again. If you get the same reaction, stop that supplement or tea altogether.

Q: I have grass allergies and can't drink red clover tea. What can I substitute for it?

A: If you are allergic to red clover tea, drink hot water and fresh lemon when you wake up in the morning to help the kidneys and liver release impurities. You can also drink one cup of dandelion root tea daily.

Q: I am experiencing die-off symptoms from detoxifying. Is this normal?

A: Yes. Many years' worth of accumulated toxins will be releasing from the body, and elimination pathways need to be supported. If you initially experience symptoms such as a headache, fatigue, achy joints, or nausea, or feel like you are getting a cold or flu, this is a normal detox response that will pass after a week or two.

Q: Is there something I can take to reduce die-off symptoms?

A: First make sure that you are eliminating the bowels daily. If you are constipated, you will recirculate toxins and feel worse. Remedies for constipation are ground flaxseed (1 or 2 tablespoons daily), magnesium citrate, triphala, probiotics, or aloe ferox. Second, drink a lot of water throughout the day. Last, you can decrease the amount of Candida abX, Gallbladder abX, and red clover tea you use. There is no rush to get up to full dosages. You might need a full week of only taking one pill or drinking one cup of red clover tea before increasing the dose. You have the option to add molybdenum or sarsaparilla. Chelated molybdenum will bind with fungal endotoxins such as acetaldehyde, making you less symptomatic. Sarsaparilla pills or tincture can also help with die-off symptoms because sarsaparilla binds with endotoxins from bacteria and yeast. If you have a headache that just won't lift, don't suffer; take an aspirin or ibuprofen if you need to take the edge off.

Q: Can I see positive results from only following the anti-candida diet and not adding the supplements to detoxify?

A: You will see marginal results if all you do is the anti-candida diet—but those results will not be long-lasting. To experience major improvements, it is essential to add herbal antimicrobials to clear out years of infection and inflammation in the body, along with other recommended supplementation to help detoxify and balance the body.

Q: Do I need to do a heavy metal detox or get rid of my mercury amalgam fillings before I start your program?

A: No. The red clover tea will chelate out heavy metals. NanoGreens10, a superfood powder I recommend the second month that contains spirulina and chlorella, will also remove heavy metals in the body.

Unless a silver amalgam filling is cracked, I don't feel those fillings need to be removed. If you have fillings wearing down and they need to be removed, I suggest replacing them with a composite filling. Make sure to wear a mask and dental dam when fillings are being drilled out; mercury is extremely toxic. For those with an autoimmune disease, especially multiple sclerosis or another neurological disorder, it's worth investigating removing silver amalgam fillings.

Q: How important is fiber in eliminating candida, and what are the best sources?

A: Fiber is the indigestible portion of plant foods, which can be soluble or insoluble; it helps control blood sugar, supports heart and gut health, and regulates bowel elimination. My favorite fiber sources are from eating green leafy vegetables, nuts/seeds, gluten-free grains, and fruit. Many people don't like to eat an array of vegetables, so I suggest 1 or 2 tablespoons of organic ground flaxseed daily to increase fiber intake and improve elimination. Chia seed and psyllium seed are other sources of fiber; since they expand in size once ingested with liquid, they can also result in some bloating and constipation, so you will have to test them out and see how they make you feel. I suggest psyllium for those experiencing diarrhea. For some people, psyllium can also alleviate constipation.

Testing and Miscellaneous

Q: I have SIBO (small intestinal bacterial overgrowth). Do I need to treat this first before doing your program?

A: Not necessarily. I feel SIBO stems from SIFO, small intestinal fungal overgrowth. The majority of people have dysbiosis, an imbalance of good to bad bacteria. It is a given to me that people will also have bacterial overgrowth, parasites, and yeast overgrowth. My 90-day program will address most infections. The typical treatment for SIBO is antibiotics, which will give temporary relief but then promote more yeast overgrowth. If you treat SIBO with antibiotics, wait to start your 90-day program until you have finished your antibiotics.

Q: Can I take diatomaceous earth (DE)?

A: Diatomaceous earth is composed of silicon dioxide (silica) from the outer shells of small single-celled plants called diatoms. I have not personally integrated DE into my practice. I don't feel there is any harm in using it, but it is not necessary. You can experience die-off symptoms when using it, and may need to cut recommended dosages in half if your symptoms don't let up.

Q: What tests are there for leaky gut, and do I need to spend the money on them?

A: No, I do not feel you need to spend the money on testing for leaky gut. Cyrex Laboratories' test markers for leaky gut are zonulin, a hormone that opens up the tight junctions between intestinal cells; lipopolysaccharides, endotoxins produced by pathogenic bacteria; and actomyosin, a protein complex that forms the contractile filaments of muscle tissue and that, when elevated, can signify that leaky gut damage is occurring. I feel there is a range of severity in leaky gut cases, and that these tests have not been perfected. In my opinion, almost everyone is dealing with some form of leaky gut, but the 90-day program should address it.

Q: I have insomnia. What can I do?

A: Quality sleep is essential to heal the body and age with quality. Your body makes physiological repairs from 10:00 p.m. to 2:00 a.m., and psychological repairs from 2:00 a.m. to 6:00 a.m. Even if you can't go to sleep at 10:00, try to lie down by 10:30 p.m. It is better to wake up earlier than to go to bed later. Make sure your bedroom is as dark as possible when you're asleep, to allow your pineal gland to secrete melatonin, and sleep with your head facing north: the best magnet is the earth itself, and sleeping head north will balance your body's magnetic field. Turn your TV off an hour before going to bed. If you need some stimuli, put on pleasant music or listen to a relaxation/sleep app. Some over-the-counter remedies I recommend for insomnia are chamomile tea steeped for twenty minutes and supplements such as Tranquil Sleep by Natural Factors and Deep Sleep by Herbs Etc.

Q: Is exercise essential while doing your program?

A: No, but it is always best to incorporate some exercise each week. Walking four to five times a week, yoga, cycling, playing a sport, or even marching in place for fifteen minutes a day while watching your favorite TV show will do. Exercise increases circulation, moves waste out of the lymphatic-immune system, helps with weight loss, increases endorphins, and promotes positive mood and quality sleep. If you are too tired the first week of your program, however, don't push it—rest and use lymphatic skin brushing to increase circulation and rid the toxins from your body.

Q: I completed my 90-day program two years ago, and my bad habits have gradually crept back in. What do I do?

A: Go back and do month one and possibly month two to get back on track.

ACKNOWLEDGMENTS

I am deeply grateful to everyone who helped me create this book. I would like to give special thanks to:

My wonderful agents, Dado Derviskadic and Steve Troha, who made my dream come true.

Karen Rinaldi and the amazing Harper Wave team . . .

My amazing editor, Julie Will, for your leadership, patience, and support.

Hudson Perigo, for your editing, inspiration, and insight.

A special thank-you to my original team: Patricia Spadaro, Nigel Yorwerth, Janet Chaikin, Bob Tinnon, and Rena.

This book would not be possible without the pioneering work of the late C. Orian Truss, MD, and William Crook, MD.

Thank you to Dr. David Perlmutter and Ann Louise Gittleman for being great supporters and believing in my work from the beginning.

To those who contributed their experiences—Anne, Charlie, Christine, Irina, Janet, Jim, Dan, Lori, Meghan, Tom, Gary, Susan, Deb, Carla, Teresa, Albert, Laura, and Leslie—thank you.

And finally, thank you to my friends and family, who are very dear to me and have always supported me along the journey: Jasmine, Perry, Steven, Irene, Josh, and my mother, who has never wavered in her loving support and is my biggest cheerleader!

RESOURCES

Supplements and Other Products

abX products, from Quintessential Healing
http://www.annboroch.com/products/
Adaptocrine, Adrenal abX, Candida abX, Gallbladder abX, Gluco abX, Glysen, Liver abX, RepairVite (K-63, caramel flavor), Thyroid abX

Bio-Design
(800) 822-6193 (say you were referred by Ann Boroch)
Aloe Lite, Aloe 225

Custom Probiotics
http://www.customprobiotics.com
11-Strain Probiotic Powder

Dr. Schulze's Original Clinical Formulae
http://www.herbdoc.com
Super-C Plus, powder or tablets

Emerson Ecologics
High-grade professional line of vitamins, supplements, and herbs.
https://wellevate.me/ann-boroch/#/patient/registration/1/17d848e08c15dd15e
6a4998e65f847
or call 800-654-4432 and ask to be signed up to wellevate under Ann Boroch
BioPharma Scientific, Designs for Health Douglas Laboratories, Innate Response, Klaire Labs, and Priority One brands

General Ecology, Inc.
http://www.generalecology.com/products.php
(800) 441-8166
Water filtration systems, including a portable system using structured matrix technology

Ionic Researchers Association
http://www.annboroch.com/products/
Ionic S.P.A. footbath

Long Life Unlimited
http://www.longlifeunlimited.com
(877) 433-3962
Aclare air purifier

Mendocino Medicinal
http://www.mendocinomedicinal.com
(707) 459-2101
Tri-Kelp (sea cabbage, bull kelp, palm kelp), a source of iodine to help maintain healthy thyroid function and to offset negative effects of radiation and heavy-metal buildup in the body. Consume ¼ to ½ teaspoon daily in a smoothie or with food. Mendocino also supplies topical compounds for pain and skin afflictions.

Mountain Rose Herbs
http://www.mountainroseherbs.com
(800) 879-3337
Organic bulk herbs: dandelion root, hibiscus, red clover dried herb, pau d'arco, chamomile, peppermint

Vitamin Warehouses
These online warehouses sell vitamins, food, and natural body-care products at reduced prices.
http://www.vitacost.com
http://www.amazon.com
http://www.iherb.com
Bio-Design, BioPharma Scientific, Biotics Research, Bob's Red Mill, Carlson, Christopher's, Designs for Health, Douglas Laboratories, Essential Formulas, Enzymedica, Gaia Herbs, Garden of Life, George's, HealthForce Nutritionals, Himalaya USA, Jarrow Formulas, Life Extension, Lily of the Desert, Klaire Labs, Made in USA, Metagenics, Nature's Way, Nordic Naturals, NOW Foods, Planetary Herbals, Priority One, Rainbow Light, ReNew Life, Solaray, and Source Naturals brands

Manufacturers and Suppliers of Specialty Foods and Beverages

The majority of products I recommend can be ordered on amazon.com, vitacost.com, and iherb.com, or by going directly to the manufacturers' websites, including those listed below, if you cannot find them in your local health food store.

Awesome Foods
http://www.awesomefoods.com
Raw breads and chips

Basiltops
http://www.basiltops.com
Dairy-free spicy and non-spicy pestos

Bragg
http://www.bragg.com
Unfermented, non-GMO soy sauce; kelp seasoning; and stevia-sweetened beverages

Coconut Secret
http://www.coconutsecret.com
Raw Coconut Aminos, Raw Coconut Flour

Food for Life
http://www.foodforlife.com
Brown and black rice tortillas

Go Raw
http://www.goraw.com
Cereals, chips, crackers, nuts, and seeds

Jilz Snackerz
http://www.jilzsnackerz.com
Jilz Gluten Free Crackerz

Just Poppin
http://www.justpoppin.com
Tru-Pop Popping Sorghum

Lydia's Organics
http://www.lydiasorganics.com
Raw breads, cereals, chips, and crackers

Majestic Garlic
http://www.majesticgarlic.com/index.php
Garlic spreads in various flavors

Mauk Family Farms
http://www.maukfamilyfarms.com
Flax crackers and crusts

Nut Just a Cookie
http://www.nutjustacookie.com
Nutty Nibbles cookies; choose sugar-free varieties

Rox Chox
http://www.roxchox.blogspot.com/p/all-about-rox-chox.html
Organic chocolate treats made with raw cacao and coconut sweetened with xylitol

Sea Tangle Noodle Company
http://www.kelpnoodles.com/index.html
Kelp noodles

Steve's PaleoGoods
http://www.stevespaleogoods.com
Steve's Original Paleo Stix (grass-fed beef sticks)

Thrive Market
http://www.thrivemarket.com
Membership for healthy foods and products at wholesale prices

Two Moms in the Raw/Soul Sprout
http://www.soulsprout.com/shop/crackers/
Sprouted almond crackers

Books on Candida

Crook, William G., MD. *The Yeast Connection: A Medical Breakthrough*. New York: Vintage, 1986.

______. *The Yeast Connection Handbook*. Garden City Park, NY: Square One, 2007.

______. *Yeast Connection Success Stories: A Collection of Stories from People Who Are Winning the Battle against Devastating Illness*. Garden City Park, NY: Square One, 2007.

Crook, William G., MD, with Elizabeth B. Crook and Hyla Cass. *The Yeast Connection and Women's Health*. Garden City Park, NY: Square One, 2007.

Kaufmann, Doug A. *The Fungus Link to Health Problems*. Rockwall, TX: MediaTrition, 2010.

Perlmutter, David, MD. *BrainRecovery.com: Powerful Therapy for Challenging Brain Disorders*. Naples, FL: Perlmutter Health Center, 2000.

______. *Grain Brain: The Surprising Truth about Wheat, Carbs, and Sugar—Your Brain's Silent Killers*. Boston: Little, Brown, 2013.

Perlmutter, David, MD, and Alberto Villoldo, PhD. *Power Up Your Brain*. Carlsbad, CA: Hay House, 2012.

Trowbridge, John P., MD, and Morton Walker, DPM. *The Yeast Syndrome: How to Help Your Doctor Identify and Treat the Real Cause of Your Yeast-Related Illness*. New York: Bantam, 1986.

Truss, C. Orian, MD. *The Missing Diagnosis*. Birmingham, AL: Missing Diagnosis, 1985.

———. *The Missing Diagnosis II*. Birmingham, AL: Missing Diagnosis, 2009.

Cookbooks

Follow your "Foods to Eat" list, as there are differences in what some candida and allergy books do and don't allow. You can also do an Internet search by typing in "candida recipes" and find many free recipes. Make sure to alter ingredients to match your "Foods to Eat" list.

Boroch, Ann, CNC. *The Candida Cure Cookbook*. Quintessential Healing, 2016.

Connolly, Pat, and Price-Pottenger Nutrition Foundation. *The Candida Albicans Yeast-Free Cookbook: How Good Nutrition Can Help Fight the Epidemic of Yeast-Related Diseases*. 2d ed. New York: McGraw-Hill, 2000.

Crook, William G., MD, and Marge H. Jones, RN. *The Yeast Connection*

Cookbook: A Guide to Good Nutrition and Better Health. Garden City Park, NY: Square One, 2007.

Greenberg, Ronald, MD, and Angela Nori. *Freedom from Allergy Cookbook*. Boulder, CO: Blue Poppy, 2000.

Jones, Marjorie H., RN. *The Allergy Self-Help Cookbook*. New York: Rodale, 2001.

Martin, Jeanne Marie, and Zoltan P. Rona. *Complete Candida Yeast Guidebook: Everything You Need to Know about Prevention, Treatment and Diet*. Rev. 2d ed. Roseville, CA: Prima Health, 2000.

Turner, Kristina. *The Self-Healing Cookbook: Whole Foods to Balance Body, Mind and Moods*. Rev. ed. Grass Valley, CA: Earthtones, 2002.

Magazines on Nutrition and Health

Life Extension (monthly; also a supplement company), www.lifeextensionretail.com

Townsend Letter (monthly), www.townsendletter.com, (360) 385-6021

Well Being Journal (published 6 times a year), www.wellbeingjournal.com, (775) 887-1702

Natural Health and Advocacy Websites

These natural health newsletters and websites provide information on nutrition, supplements, advocacy, and natural solutions for healing.

www.anh-usa.org (Alliance for Natural Health)
www.livestrong.com
www.mercola.com
www.naturalcures.com
www.naturalnews.com
www.organicconsumers.org (Organic Consumers Association)
www.price-pottenger.org (Price-Pottenger Nutrition Foundation)
www.thenhf.com (National Health Federation)

Books and Resources on Mind-Body Healing

Byrne, Rhonda. *The Secret*. DVD. Prime Time Productions, 2006. http://www.thesecret.tv/index.html.

Chopra, Deepak. *Quantum Healing: Exploring the Frontiers of Mind/Body Medicine*. New York: Bantam, 1990.

Dwoskin, Hale. *The Sedona Method: Your Key to Lasting Happiness, Success, Peace and Emotional Well-Being*. Sedona, 2003.

Emotional Freedom Technique, http://www.emofree.com. This therapeutic technique helps you to release fears, phobias, addictions, cravings, and fear-based and negative thoughts and emotions.

Hay, Louise L. *You Can Heal Your Life*. Carlsbad, CA: Hay House, 1999.

Kasl, Charlotte. *If the Buddha Got Stuck: A Handbook for Change on a Spiritual Path*. New York: Penguin, 2005.

Lipton, Bruce H. *The Biology of Belief: Unleashing the Power of Consciousness, Matter, and Miracles*. Carlsbad, CA: Hay House, 2008.

Maté, Gabor, MD. *When the Body Says No: Exploring the Stress-Disease Connection*. Hoboken, NJ: Wiley, 2011.

Myss, Caroline, PhD. *Anatomy of the Spirit*. New York: Three Rivers Press, 1997.

Pert, Candace B. *Molecules of Emotion: The Science behind Mind-Body Medicine*. New York: Touchstone, 1997.

Siegel, Bernie S. *Love, Medicine and Miracles*. New York: Random House, 1999.

Sincero, Jen. *You Are a Badass: How to Stop Doubting Your Greatness and Start Living an Awesome Life*. Philadelphia: Running Press, 2013.

Spadaro, Patricia. *Honor Yourself: The Inner Art of Giving and Receiving*. Bozeman, MT: Three Wings, 2009.

Tolle, Eckhart. *The Power of Now: A Guide to Spiritual Enlightenment*. San Francisco: New World Library, 2004.

Wilde, Stuart. *Infinite Self: 33 Steps to Reclaiming Your Inner Power*. Carlsbad, CA: Hay House, 1996.

Health Documentaries

Bought (2014)
The Business of Disease (2014)
A Delicate Balance: The Truth (2008)
Doctored (2012)
Fast Food Nation (2006)
Fat, Sick & Nearly Dead (2010)
Food, Inc. (2008)
Food Matters (2008)

Fresh (2009)
The Future of Food (2004)
Genetic Roulette: The Gamble of Our Lives (2012)
Hungry for Change (2013)
King Corn: You Are What You Eat (2007)
Processed People (2009)
Unacceptable Levels (2012)

Laboratories

Cyrex Laboratories
www.cyrexlabs.com
(602) 759-1245
Multi-tissue antibody testing for autoimmune conditions, gluten intolerance, and cross-reactivity food sensitivities

Diagnos-Techs
www.diagnostechs.com
(206) 251-0596
Salivary hormonal testing

Direct Labs
www.directlabs.com
(800) 908-0000
Provides blood chemistry panels, including the Apex 4 panel (a full blood chemistry panel with a vitamin D test), without a doctor's prescription

Genova Diagnostics
www.gdx.net
(800) 522-4762
Stool and blood testing for candida, parasites, and gluten intolerance

NOTES

Chapter 1: The Candida Epidemic

1. Jane Peterson et al., "The NIH Microbiome Project," *Genome Research* 19, no. 12 (December 2009): 2317–23.
2. Lijia Cui, Alison Morris, Elodie Ghedin Cui, et al., "The Mycobiome in Health and Disease," *Genome Medicine* 5, no. 63 (July 2013), https://genomemedicine.biomedcentral.com/articles/.
3. Mahmoud Ghannoum, "The Mycobiome," *Scientist*, February 2016, http://www.the-scientist.com/?articles.view/articleNo/45153/title/The-Mycobiome/.
4. Gary B. Huffnagle and Mairi C. Noverr, "The Emerging World of the Fungal Microbiome," *Trends in Microbiology* 21, no. 7 (July 2013): 334–41.
5. //www.cdc.gov/media/releases/2016/p0503-unnecessary-prescriptions.html.
6. http://www.webmd.com/a-to-z-guides/news/20150417/superbugs-what-they-are#1, https://www.nytimes.com/2017/02/27/health/who-bacteria-pathogens-antibiotic-resistant-superbugs.html.
7. S. Leclercq, F. M. Mian, et al., "Low-Dose Penicillin in Early Life Induces Long-Term Changes in Gut Microbiota, Brain Cytokines, and Behavior," *Nature Communications* 8 (April 4, 2017): 15062.
8. Arielle Nagler, MD, et al., "The Use of Oral Antibiotics before Isotretinoin Therapy in Patients with Acne," *Journal of the American Academy of Dermatology* 74, no. 2 (February 2016): 273–79.
9. A. Pierron et al., "Impact of Two Mycotoxins, Deoxynivalenol and Fumonisin, on Pig Intestinal Health," *Porcine Health Management* 2, no. 21 (September 2016).
10. Michael J. Kennedy and Paul A. Volz, "Ecology of *Candida albicans* Gut Colonization: Inhibition of Candida Adhesion, Colonization, and Dissemination from the Gastrointestinal Tract by Bacterial Antagonism," *Infection and Immunity* 49, no. 3 (September 1985): 654–63.
11. Ibid., 659.
12. X. Zhang et al., "Estrogen Effects on *Candida albicans*: A Potential Virulence-Regulating Mechanism," *Journal of Infectious Disease* 181, no. 4 (April 2000): 1441–46.

13. G. G. Donders et al., "Management of Recurrent Vulvo-Vaginal Candidosis as a Chronic Illness," *Gynecologic and Obstetric Investigation* 70, no. 4 (2010): 306–21.
14. http://authors.library.caltech.edu/72032/.
15. http:www.neurology.org/content/88/21/1996.
16. Diana Pisa et al., "Different Brain Regions Are Infected with Fungi in Alzheimer's Disease," *Nature Online Scientific Reports* 5, no. 15015 (2015).
17. Emily G. Severance et al., "*Candida albicans* Exposures, Sex Specificity and Cognitive Deficits in Schizophrenia and Bipolar Disorder," *NPJ Schizophrenia* 4, no. 2 (May 4, 2016): 16018.
18. https://www.ncbi.nlm.nih.gov/pmc/articles/PMC4069141/.
19. Ed Silverman, "Why Did Prescription Spending Hit $374B in the US Last Year?" *Wall Street Journal*, April 14, 2015.

Chapter 2: The Origin of Disease

1. Iurii Koboziev et al., "Gut-Associated Lymphoid Tissue, T-Cell Trafficking, and Chronic Intestinal Inflammation," *Annals of the New York Academy of Sciences* 1207, suppl. 1 (October 2010): E86–93.
2. Michael Karin et al., "Innate Immunity Gone Awry: Linking Microbial Infections to Chronic Inflammation and Cancer," *Cell* 124, no. 4 (February 24, 2006): 823–35.
3. Carol A. Kumamoto, "Inflammation and Gastrointestinal Candida Colonization," *Current Opinion in Microbiology* 14, no. 4 (August 2011): 386–91.
4. A. Louveau, I. Smirnov, T. J. Keyes, J. D. Eccles, S. J. Rouhani, J. D. Peske, N. C. Derecki, D. Castle, J. W. Mandell, K. S. Lee, T. H. Harris, and J. Kipnis, "Structural and Functional Features of Central Nervous System Lymphatic Vessels," *Nature* 523, June 1, 2015, doi: 10.1038/nature14432. [Epub ahead of print.] PMID: 26030524.

Chapter 3: Using the Mind to Help Heal the Body

1. Michael Speca et al., "A Randomized, Wait-List Controlled Clinical Trial: The Effect of a Mindfulness Meditation-Based Stress Reduction Program on Mood and Symptoms of Stress in Cancer Outpatients," *Psychosomatic Medicine* 62 (2000): 613–22.
2. Sat Bir S. Khalsa et al., "Evaluation of the Mental Health Benefits of Yoga in a Secondary School: A Preliminary Randomized Controlled Trial," *Journal of Behavioral Health Sciences and Research*, June 2, 2011.

Chapter 4: Candida Detox

1. John P. Trowbridge and Morton Walker, *The Yeast Syndrome: How to Help Your Doctor Identify and Treat the Real Cause of Your Yeast-Related Illness* (New York: Bantam, 1986), 129.

Chapter 5: Starve the Yeast, Nourish Your Body

1. https://www.ncbi.nlm.nih.gov/pubmed/27601306.
2. https://www.ncbi.nlm.nih.gov/pubmed/27215959.
3. M. C. Lomer, G. C. Parkes, and J. D. Sanderson, "Lactose Intolerance in Clinical Practice—Myths and Realities," *Alimentary Pharmacology and Therapies* 27, no. 2 (January 2008): 93–103.
4. Maura Keller, "Food Intolerances vs. Food Allergies," *Today's Dietitian* 13, no. 10 (October 2011): 52.
5. W. F. Nieuwenhuizen et al., "Is *Candida albicans* a Trigger in the Onset of Coeliac Disease?" *Lancet* 361, no. 9375 (June 2003).
6. Marios Hadjivassiliou et al., "Gluten Sensitivity: From Gut to Brain," *Lancet Neurology* 9, no. 3 (March 2010): 318–30.
7. Fereydoon Batmanghelidj, *Your Body's Many Cries for Water* (Falls Church, VA: Global Health Solutions, 1995), 69.
8. Fereydoon Batmanghelidj, *Water for Health, for Healing, for Life: You're Not Sick, You're Thirsty!* (New York: Warner, 2003), 185.

INDEX

ABOUT THE AUTHOR

Ann Boroch was a certified nutritional consultant and naturopath, as well as an educator and speaker on the topics of nutrition, naturopathy, allergies, autoimmune diseases, gastrointestinal health, and candida. Ann authored two books, *Healing Multiple Sclerosis* and *The Candida Cure*, and for more than twenty years maintained a practice in Los Angeles, where she treated thousands of patients back to optimum health. Ann passed away in 2017, shortly after finishing her work on the revised edition of *The Candida Cure*.

For more information, contact:
www.annboroch.com